FUEL AND FIRE

Dominate Obstacle Course Racing
With Scientific Training Strategies
Fueled By Nutrition

MIKE DEIBLER

outskirts
press

TABLE OF CONTENTS

Introduction   i

Acknowledgements   ix

Chapter 1: How to Use This Book   1

Chapter 2: The Assessments   4

Chapter 3: Recovery   18

Chapter 4: Endurance   32

Chapter 5: Cardiorespiratory Workouts   38

Chapter 6: Strength Training   48

Chapter 7: Tactical Training   139

Chapter 8: Nutrition   151

Chapter 9: Mental Training   165

Chapter 10: Get to Work   173

Appendix: Training Plan   177

Works Cited   183

INTRODUCTION

Congratulations! You have taken a huge step toward learning better, more evidence-based ways to enhance your health and performance.

There are many reasons that could have brought you to this moment. You may be searching to improve your training and nutrition. You may be new to obstacle course racing (OCR) and want to understand how to approach the sport. Perhaps you've raced for years and are struggling to break through a plateau. Maybe you are frustrated by illness and injury and the health you need to train and race eludes you.

Whatever the reason is, I have answers for you.

ARE YOU READY?

Before we begin, I must ask you this: Are you ready? You are, right? My intention is to take you on a journey. The Hero's Journey.

The Hero's Journey consists of three stages including Departure, Initiation, and Return. In the Departure, the hero is living in an ordinary world but is called to go on an adventure. The Initiation involves the hero traveling into the unknown, where he or she faces trials, challenges, and tasks. In this stage the hero overcomes a major challenge or obstacle, walking away a different person. Then, finally, our hero goes through The Return. The Return is where the hero traverses back to the ordinary world a changed person -- having gained knowledge or power in order to help others.

Sounds familiar right? You can plug in just about any movie or book and see the journey. Star Wars offers a vivid example.

But this is not a fantasy or science fiction novel you are reading. While I am not asking you to save the world, I am asking you to journey into the unknown. I am telling you now that you will encounter challenge and struggle. No one likes to change. No one likes to do things differently. This is why many get stuck in frustration, failing to see their hard work pay off.

But if you are ready, I am here to help you with the process. I want to show you a few things I have learned over the years I know will help.

It's a process you must trust, though. I am asking you to take a leap of faith. I am also asking you to put in a thorough effort. To do the work. Many will read this book and take away only fragments, bits and pieces, of what I designed to be a complete system. A system that works best as a whole. So, let's dive in. Let's start our adventure.

OCR is an amazing sport. Whether you are doing it for more recreation or competition, it has something in it for everyone. It will challenge you endlessly. But when you cross the finish line, you are hooked.

This is your chance to prove to yourself what you are made of and give yourself the satisfaction of an accomplishment most are too afraid to try. Racing alone isn't enough, however. You to push yourself harder, press against the limits and discover the next level.

The great thing about OCR is that it evens the playing field for different types of athletes. You need endurance; you need to be a runner; you need strength, power, agility, balance, and many other bio-motor capacities. You need to be ready for anything.

There are great runners that get hung up on the obstacles and there are great strength athletes that get slowed by the running and rough terrain. Specialization will cost you. You must strive for mastery of different domains.

This unique aspect of OCR makes it more enjoyable to train for. You will not be spending your time on one specific area. You may focus more on certain weaknesses, but you must have a balanced approach in your training.

You must also take this approach with your fueling and nutrition. There are different ways the body will generate and recycle energy. We often assume that whatever we eat we breakdown and turn into fuel. The body can only use certain fuels at certain times based on the type of activity you are doing. Your goal is to be as efficient as possible and quickly switch between fuel sources. The human body is amazing at adapting to different stressors and different stimuli.

You will be fueling based on the needs of your body -- not simply applying a single approach to each and every day. By learning and better understanding how the body uses the fuel that you get from food and how it prefers certain foods based on the training you are doing, you gain a huge advantage over others.

The common methodology is to pick a diet like Paleo, ketogenic, Zone, high-carb, etc., and train as hard as you can. Although this combination will show some progress in the beginning, it won't yield long-term success. Progress will stall, you'll burn out, and your racing career will be a short one.

Within the pages of this book you will find answers. You will also find simple plans to follow. If you do not care about why we do certain things in our training and fueling, skip straight to the plan.

But I have a feeling -- especially since this is not a traditional, cookie-cutter plan -- you will not want to skip over the why. You have a powerful reason for reading a book like this. You want to understand the WHY behind everything. When you can understand this, your options are unlimited, and you will become unstoppable.

Allow me to explain what I mean: My goal in writing this was not just to give out a generic plan. It was to show you the way that you can develop your own plan. I want you to understand how the body works to fuel the workouts you will be pushing yourself though.

Not only that, I want you to have a long career. The direction the fitness industry is trending can be scary sometimes to see. When we look at those who have been using traditional training and traditional modalities for a significant period of time, we see all the issues they are suffering from now.

Consider how many former runners can no longer run, or are forced to have joint replacements, or have simply lost their enjoyment for running; or all the above. These consequences are unfortunately all too common in a non-contact sport that is viewed as a healthy lifestyle.

OCR's are demanding. Every time you step out to compete, you are pushing yourself harder than you may want to. You are not tip-toeing out of your comfort zone but taking a gigantic leap.

This can take a toll. If you are not working to move better, take care of your body, and fuel properly, you will quickly discover that you will not have many competitive races in you.

But -- when you train and fuel optimally -- you will enjoy your racing and training as astonished others characterize you as "age-defying."

Whether you are a first-timer, a recreational runner just trying to get through a race easier, or an elite competitor trying to podium, you will find value in this book in supporting your journey toward becoming a true OCR athlete.

ABOUT THE AUTHOR

I can remember that day back in grad school more vividly than most days. I was finally going to give up; finally getting the nerve to call my parents up and let them know I was done. I never wanted to disappoint them or myself, but it was time to quit.

Back in the fall of 2004, I was at the University of Florida going to school for my master's degree, making school my priority for a two-year period.

I had always been a great student and did very well in undergrad, but those were years (I must admit) I put my sport and training in front of my education.

I did my work and took my tests, but luckily it was something that came easily for me. I studied, went to class, and graduated with a great GPA. But track was more of my passion and took more of my focus. I do not regret this and learned so much from this experience and made incredible friends along the way.

My track career was a success. I completed my eligibility and seemed to go out on top in a John Elway-like fashion.

OK, maybe not as cool as winning a Super Bowl and then retiring, but in my final collegiate meet I finished with a personal best at the NCAA Division I championships with a high jump of 2.18m, which is just under 7 feet 2 inches.

This height was good enough for an eighth-place finish, earning All-American honors. This was one of my proudest achievements, one I still get goosebumps thinking about.

I always had a joke during my time in training. My healthiest day was the very first day of practice my freshman year. After that, it all went downhill. Sure, I attained success, but at a cost.

During my four years of competing in college I suffered countless injuries. It seemed that I spent just as much time in the athletic training room as the weight room. In my career I suffered from Achilles tendinitis, patella tendinosis, shoulder impingement, and pain in just about every other major joint of the body.

At one point I started getting incredible groin pain on one side. The pain eventually creeped into my lower abdomen, and then across to the other side of the groin. I never received a firm diagnosis on that one. I was told it was "probably tendinitis" but I had heard these words so often I had come to believe this was the standard opinion when they weren't sure what was going on.

I remember being just 21-years-old and dreading driving a car for more than 20 minutes. I would actually swing my right leg across to the passenger side and drive with my left foot because of the searing pain in my knee. On airplanes, I had to fight for an aisle seat. Sitting in the movie theater was flat-out unbearable.

If this was what my body was doing in my twenties, what did my future hold?

Despite this, when my college career was up, I moved to Florida. I wanted to focus more on school -- my master's degree program -- but I really couldn't let athletics go. So, I started to train with the university team with the intention to qualify for the US Olympic Trials. At that point I was just 2 cm away from the jump I needed to make the qualification standard.

The University of Florida was, and still is, one of the best track and field programs in the country. The training was intense and much more than I was used to. Any injuries that had started to fade came back full force.

Everything hurt all the time. I had come to realize that maybe this wasn't the best thing for me.

As I finished up my first semester, I decided to give up my dream of making the Trials. It was no longer worth it. I did not want to find out what my future would be like if I continued down this path.

I made peace with my decision and do not regret it. I finished my schooling, met the woman of my dreams, and moved to San Diego to start my career as a personal trainer and strength coach. This was work I have always enjoyed and knew I could spend my life mastering this craft.

As time went on, I picked up various sports like beach volleyball and basketball to help fill the void of competition. It was fun for a while, but nothing really seemed to stick. It wasn't until I signed up for my first Spartan Race that I really caught the bug.

After completing my first race, it was like the scratch of an itch I couldn't reach for years. I knew I had to do another one and I knew I had to figure out better ways to train for the events.

I immersed myself in the OCR world, which was all new for me. I trained hard and raced more and more. I loved it all, but started to become concerned with typical OCR training and mentality.

The idea of go hard or go home was everywhere. Don't get me wrong, I love a tough workout and challenge, but there is much more to training than trying to kill yourself, just to say you got through some crazy workout. It never made sense.

I began to see people going on the same path I went down with my training in college. Strength and conditioning have come a long way since then. We know so much more and can train in smarter ways, leading to less injuries, better performance, and longer competitive careers.

Many of the issues I dealt with earlier in life were due to poor training habits and over-training. I beat my body into the ground. I had success, but at a huge cost. And I will always wonder how much better I could have been knowing what I know now.

My goal has been to help educate others on this journey. OCR racing is an incredible sport, one we learn more and more about as it matures. I can look back at how my own personal training plan has evolved the more I learned about the sport.

I never thought I would run as much as I do right now. I still have improvements to make, but I come from an event where I took eight steps, jumped, then rested for 5-10 minutes. Never did I imagine running a race that took eight hours to complete.

But I did, and I and continue to do it without the major injuries I routinely suffered through. My body feels great. Even when I have an ache or pain pop up, I know how to take care of it, recover, and get back to work when I can.

The whole world of OCR has pushed me as an athlete and as a coach. I had to learn specifically how to become stronger and more powerful at obstacles while also becoming a runner. I never thought I would say that, but I am a runner and I have learned how to go from hating running, to tolerating it, to enjoying it.

My passion is to help others learn from my experiences. I became an SGX Coach to help others learn specifically how to train for races and obstacles. I started a podcast and website, interviewing other coaches and sharing philosophies on different ways to train and improve movement.

I want to show you not only how to maximize your performance, but how you can do it without sacrificing your body. I want to turn you into an athlete than can handle anything and have a long-lasting career in this great sport.

ACKNOWLEDGEMENTS

There are so many that have helped pave the way for me and assist in writing this book whether they know it or not. I fear that I am leaving some out, but know that I am forever grateful for the help to inspire me to write this book and give me the knowledge to share with others. Special appreciate goes to:

My wife, Emily, and Davis and Ellis

My parents

Stephanie Guitierrez

Gray Cook, Lee Burton, Brett Jones, Diane Vives, Michelle Desser and the rest of the incredible team at Functional Movement Systems

Michael Boyle

Brendon Rearick, Kevin Carr, and the Certified Functional Strength Coach Team

Dan John

Alywn and Rachel Cosgove

Brandon Marcello

Jen Rhoton

And to all of my clients who have trusted me to put these ideas into practice to help them reach their goals.

CHAPTER 1

HOW TO USE THIS BOOK

This book will not be for everyone. There are plenty of beginner guides and books that do an excellent job explaining the different types of races, obstacles, and starter workout plans. If you are looking for the basics, you will find other resources that may help you better. Rather, this book is going somewhere that no other OCR book has gone, at least not that I have seen to date.

We will take a deep dive into everything you need to consider for training purposes to not only get better for any obstacle course race, but excel. This means maximizing your training so you reach your individual peak potential, whether that is finishing an elite race, coming in the top 10%, or stepping onto that podium. In the coming pages I will hold nothing back. I reveal all the training secrets that have helped my own training as well as all of my clients.

This book is simply a guide. There is no single way to help you reach your goals. We are going to use proven methods to improve your nutrition, increase your efficiency, and dial up your training. As mentioned earlier, it is not enough to just follow a meal plan or a program. This may be a place to start, but I want more for you.

Instead, in the following pages, you will learn how to eat properly based on your training needs; how to train properly based on your performance goals; and gain an understanding in how you can continue to do this long after the program I have laid out for you is up.

This is simply your starting point. With each section you will learn a training technique that you will master and use to improve your exercise routine. You will also receive fueling lessons on nutrition.

In this book you will learn how to balance nutrition and training. But the key is consistency. It takes time to adapt to demands you are making on your body. Your body may even fight you in the beginning. Life will get in the way. I do not expect you to be perfect, but do want you to be consistent.

With consistency you should expect progress. You will be given the tools to help determine if your plan is working. You will start to register changes. Never follow a program blindly. If you are consistent and do not see the changes occur, you will understand how to tweak things based on your specific needs.

For starters, you will learn how to properly assess your current situation. Our assessment for training will help determine your areas of biggest concern. This will help you map out priorities. You will also assess your nutrition to understand what your starting point is and to get an idea of how you will track your fueling.

From here you will learn basic physiology so you understand how the workouts you will be performing tap the different energy systems of the body. This will help you determine what type of fueling needs each specific type of workout will require.

We will dissect the different areas of training that will need to be incorporated including your recovery strategies, endurance training, strength training, and tactical training. I refer to this as the R.E.S.T. system.

Each component of training is listed in order of importance. As you learn about each system you will also discover the value of each macronutrient, plus other strategies to help you implement better nutrition habits.

Next, you will learn how to put this all together into a complete and progressive exercise and nutrition plan, with practical guides and tools to help you begin.

And finally you will be given a complete plan that can operate as a template for race preparation. The template allows you to mold your Fuel and Fire program toward the goal of maximizing your performance for your next race, and future races.

With all of this, you will have all the tools needed for improved performance and -- critically -- a longer-lasting racing career.

CHAPTER 2

THE ASSESSMENTS

As mentioned earlier, one of the attractive things about OCR's is the fact that you need to excel at several different tasks. In order to get started with our training you must understand how to assess your current abilities with each of these tasks. Once you have an idea of where your strengths and weaknesses are you can better determine priorities.

You can go overboard with different assessments and based on your situation you may need a more specialized eye to help you along the way. For the purposes of this book we will focus on the basic assessments that you can do on your own or with the assistance of a friend.

Let's look at each of the components we will need to train and how we can assess them.

MOVEMENT

Your capability with movement can be a hard thing to assess, an area athletes will often skip over. For the purposes of this book the topic of movement screening is too large to cover. So instead we will discuss why assessing the quality of your movement is imperative and direct you to a resource.

On the wave of excitement that comes with starting a new exercise program, many want to jump right in and push to their limits.

But what are your limits?

A key question to answer at the outset: Do you move well enough to train for the physical demands of an OCR?

OCR's will require a lot of your body. If you cannot move with minimum capacity, it's a matter of time before your body will break down and let you know about it.

You at least need the basic movement patterns down. This includes squatting, lunging, single leg stance, lifting, pushing, pulling, and rotating.

We are not requiring perfect movement; instead we want to see if you can perform these movement patterns without pain and without unnecessary compensations. This is your basic movement screen.

Think of when you go to the doctor for a regular checkup. One of your vital signs the doctor will always check is your blood pressure. If the reading is normal, your doctor will check the box and go to the next test. There is no need to be concerned with anything regarding blood pressure. Now if you get record an abnormally high blood pressure level, further testing will be required to decide the best course of action.

The movement screen is checking your vital signs for movement. If everything looks adequate you can move on. But if it does not -- and most people have at least one issue here -- then it is appropriate to look at your movement quality further to decide the best course of action.

A great resource for this is the Functional Movement Screen (FMS). You will need a trained coach to take you through the screen, but it is worth the small investment to improve movement quality. The FMS looks at 7 movement patterns and scores you on how your perform each. Visit www.functionalmovement.com to find a coach near you. We will latter discuss the Fundamental Capacity Screen which looks to see if you have minimum capacities for more performance measures.

After completing a screen you will know what movement patterns you are cleared to train and what patterns you will need to work on and improve. Once you clear the movement screen by checking all the boxes, you are good to go. This is the cornerstone of your program. Otherwise you will start your way down the dark path of injury and compensation. It won't be a matter of if but of when, and can be hard to come back from.

While finding a professional to screen your movement is always the best option, you can perform a self-screen to get an idea if this is an area of concern or not. While I could explain this screen in this text, I will send you a free bonus for purchasing this book.

Visit https://ocrunderground.com/ocr-self-screening-tests/ to receive a free self screening guide to follow.

POWER

The ability to generate, use, and absorb power is an integral piece of your racing. If you are trying to sprint up a hill, jump over or down from a wall, or throw a spear, you will be relying on your body's capacity to generate power.

There are several different tests we can use to judge your power development for both the upper and lower body. To save time, yet still net a great deal of information, we will pick simple tests you can perform easily at home. The information will suggest if where more work is needed.

For power, we are going to use the standing broad jump. You will perform two variations of this test to get the most you can out of it. While the broad jump is a classic lower-body power development assessment, you are also looking at how the upper body is contributing to generating force.

For our testing you will perform a standing broad jump using your arms first. You will take the best of three attempts. To start this test, you will need a tape measure. Lay out the tape measure first. Start with your toes lined up on the zero mark.

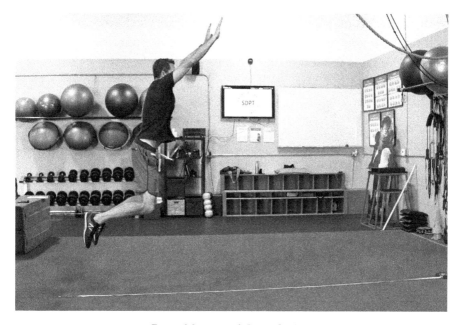

Broad Jump w/ Arm Swing

You will perform a max distance countermovement jump by squatting down and reaching your arms behind you. Then explode out and swing your arms up, with the arms reaching as far as you can. For the jump to count you must stick the landing so you can measure where your heels are against the tape measure.

If feet are not even, you will take the distance from the closest heel to the start, using inches or centimeters.

Repeat for three attempts.

Your goal is to be able to jump at least your height. So if you are 5 feet 10 inches tall (70 inches) you will want a broad jump of more than 70 inches.

Next you will repeat the same exact test but now you will perform it with your arms on your hips. This will most likely feel awkward, but you will see how your armless jump will compare to your arm swing jump. Test in the same fashion taking the best of three.

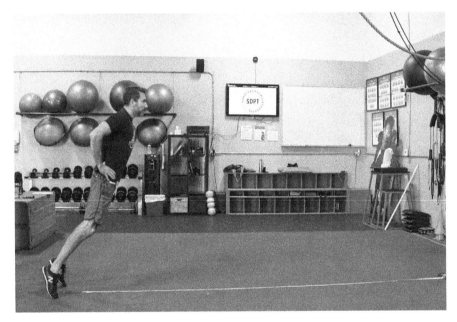

Broad Jump w/ No Arm Swing

Your jump with no arm swing should be no more than 20% less than your jump with hands. If there is too much of a difference it means you are using your upper body without full contribution of the lower body. This means we will have to focus on improving the lower body's ability to generate power. If your armless jump is equal to your with arm jump, then we need to work on the upper body contribution.

STRENGTH

Strength is a necessity for OCR training and racing. You will need to be strong enough to lift and carry things. Traditionally 1 Rep Max (1RM) Testing is used to determine strength levels and these may be appropriate.

This type of assessment comes with a higher risk of injury so caution should be taken. If you decide to perform 1RM Testing, make sure you own the movement you are testing and are safe. We will cover other movements in the strength training portion of this book. For assessment purposes, we will not look at every movement, but instead your ability to maintain integrity under load.

For the majority of assessments, I prefer to use another technique used in the Fundamental Capacity Screen (FCS). While it is not necessarily a strength test, I like to throw it in the category. This would be a postural control screen. You have likely seen or experienced this as a farmer's carry.

Based off the research from the FCS, we will use 75% of your body weight split between each arm. You can use dumbbells, kettlebells, sandbags, or anything else that you can carry in each hand.

To perform this test, you will set up two cones 25-feet apart. Place the weights at the start line next to one of the cones. You will both time this drill as well as measure total distance covered. When ready you will pick up the weights. It will be easier to have a partner with you to start a timer when you begin walking.

Execute this test walking with a tall posture, creating a figure eight pattern around the two cones. When you can no longer hold the weight securely, you stop the test. Be honest here. If there is any change in posture or grip, you will stop. Whatever grip you start with you must stay with for the entire test.

For this test you will track both your distance traveled and your time that you held on. Your goal is to hold for a minimum of 90 seconds and travel 250 feet.

GRIP STRENGTH

It goes without saying but grip strength is going to be critical to your success in racing. The farmer's carry is one way to test grip strength, although it is evaluating other capacities as well. But grip strength has multiple dimensions you'll need to measure.

The farmer's carry is one way to examine your grip within the ability to carry something. Another important type of grip is hanging grip. When getting through monkey bars and other hanging obstacles you will need to maximize your ability to hang.

For this reason, we will also add a dead hang and flex hang test. While in the race you are not just hanging but also required to control your body during a traverse. But this will be too difficult to assess. For simplicity we will use your ability to hang from a bar as an overall indicator of grip strength. For these tests you will simply need a pull-up bar and stopwatch.

The dead hang will be measured with a clocking of your max hang time, with arms totally extended. Your goal is a minimum of 60 seconds. The flex hang is your max time with your elbows bent so your chin remains above the bar. Once your chin drops below the bar you stop the time. Your goal is to flex hang for a minimum of 30 seconds.

MUSCULAR ENDURANCE

Muscular endurance refers to the amount of repetitions a muscle or group of muscles can complete until failure.

It is clear to see the importance of having good muscular endurance for a race. Being able to get through burpees with less strain on the body, having to push or pull an object for an extended period, or being able to hang long enough to make it through monkey bars or a rig are all examples where muscular endurance is essential.

There are a few different tests to use for evaluating your muscular endurance. Many may use the max number of reps of an exercise one can do in a minute. This may be a decent indicator of endurance, but what if you need or can go longer than one minute?

Another problem with this type of test is you may just improve your speed of an exercise versus actual endurance. For example, if you were able to do 20 pushups in a minute the first time you test, and then retest and get 30, did you improve your endurance? Or did you improve your speed?

For this reason, we will test your muscular endurance by using a cadence test. You can pick a number of different exercises for this, but I think pushups or body weight squats are great selections.

For pushups, we will start with the assumption that you are doing push-ups from your toes. For this test you will need a metronome to keep a beat and a small object, like a tennis ball, to mark the lower point of the push up.

Set the metronome for 50 beats per minute. At each beat you will move through half a rep. So, starting in the top position, when you hear the first beep, lower down and touch your chest to the tennis ball. Stay there until you hear the next beep and go back to the top. Continue moving at this pace until you can no longer complete a rep or you cannot keep up with the pace. Note your number of completed reps.

If you cannot do pushups from your toes, then this test can be modified. A great place to perform this test is using a squat rack or Smith machine.

Here you can adjust a bar to any height you need to and complete the same exact test with incline pushups.

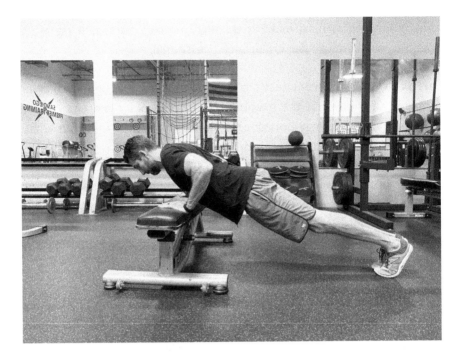

Many will just drop to their knees as a modification, but this is a completely different exercise. We will want to test from the toes, even if you modify with an incline.

We can also perform this same exact test with body weight squats. Here you will use the same metronome to 50 beats per minute. Now you just need an object to mark the lowest point reached in your squat.

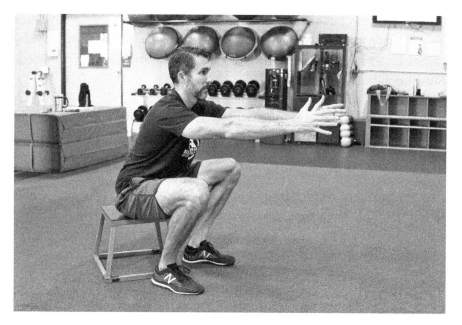

Box Squat

This will be different for everyone based on your level of mobility and ability. Find your end range for your squat and match it with an object such as a box or medicine ball. The goal should be to get your thigh parallel to the floor. Perform as many squats as possible until you can no longer complete a rep or keep up with the pace.

There are no established norms for these testing procedures to date, but personal experience says men should aim for over 20 pushups and women for over 15. For squats, men and women usually score similar numbers. Shoot for a goal of at least 40 reps.

CARDIORESPIRATORY ENDURANCE

Cardiorespiratory endurance refers to improving the efficiency between the cardiovascular system and the respiratory system. When these two systems work effectively, you will notice that long duration work seems easier and easier.

This will be the bulk of the training we will discuss in this book, since your training for a race will heavily depend on your ability to go for long distances. Other aspects of training are important, but this is where most people struggle.

For assessments we are going to focus on two different tests. These tests will include the 1.5-mile run and the 30-minute lactate threshold test.

The 1.5 mile run test is straight forward. You will run that distance as fast as you can. Make sure to start with an appropriate warm-up before-hand. Each time you retest make sure you use the same trail or course to be consistent. You will record your average pace and final time.

To get an idea of where you should be, you can check against the standards of the Cooper 1.5-mile test times. Using an app like Strava is a great way to measure your average pace, but there are many great programs out there to help you track.

Rating	Males	Females
Very Poor	> 16:01	> 19:01
Poor	16:00 - 14:01	19:00 - 18:31
Fair	14:00 - 12:01	18:30 - 15:55
Good	12:00 - 10:46	15:54 - 13:31
Excellent	10:45 - 9:45	13:30-12:30
Superior	< 9:44	< 12:29

*data from www.topendsports.com

While this is not a purely aerobic measurement, it will be a good indicator of your endurance pace and a simple exercise that you can perform at any level.

The 30-minute lactate threshold test is going to be more of a challenge. If you are new to racing you may not be ready for this type of testing, but the information it provides you is incredibly important for your training program.

We will discuss further what lactate is and why knowing your lactate threshold is so important, but for now we will simply focus on how to do the test.

Start with an easy 5-10 minute warm-up jog. When ready you will start a timer and run the fastest pace you can maintain for 30 minutes. This can be tricky. You do not want to go out too hard and not be able to maintain your speed, nor do you want to go out too slow and leave too much in the tank.

Your goal will be to maintain a relatively constant pace for the entire trial. At 10 minutes you will note your heart rate (HR). Then at the completion of the test you will again note your HR. Take the average HR between those two numbers. This will be your lactate threshold heart rate.

Assuming you kept a constant pace, you will also track your average pace for the run. Both numbers will be important for determining your training run intensities.

GRIT

Let's face it. You are going to have to do things you do not want to do. This will be true for your training, nutrition, and racing. Some are willing to accept this and push through. Others will back off and not accept the challenge.

While grit is something very difficult to assess or put a number on, we are going to have you do something you probably don't want to do.

This will be your 5-minute burpee test. It will be performed just like it sounds. How many complete burpees can you perform in 5 minutes?

This is a tough test and there will be points when you will want to give up. But, do you have what it takes? First step is simply performing the test. But the real challenge is, can you push yourself during this test? Can you get every last burpee out of you in 5 minutes?

If you need motivation, you can use the chart below to pick a goal to aim for. This is the Spartan Fitness Challenge score sheet.

MEN						
Age	14-19	20-29	30-39	40-49	50-59	60+
Hire a Coach	<53	<55	<53	<48	<45	<40
Do More Burpees	53	55	53	48	45	40
Healthy	68	70	68	63	60	55
Spartan Fit	83	85	83	78	75	70

Women						
Age	14-19	20-29	30-39	40-49	50-59	60+
Hire a Coach	<43	<50	<45	<40	<37	<32
Do More Burpees	43	50	45	40	37	32
Healthy	58	65	60	55	52	47
Spartan Fit	73	80	75	70	67	62

*data from www.spartancoaches.com

TURN WEAKNESSES INTO STRENGTHS

I have given you a great deal of information to start with. This will guide you in the right direction to learn more about yourself and what you need to focus on. We tend to want to focus on the things we are good at. While it is important to train all aspects of fitness, we must pay special attention to where we struggle.

We need to accept the idea that we are going to do things we really do not want to do. But this is what will truly get you stronger.

Now that you know where your strengths and weakness are you can determine how much time is needed in each phase and style of training. In the next section we will cover the essentials to your training program.

As you go through your training it is good to reassess. You may not have to redo all the previously discussed tests, but pick one or two of your biggest trouble areas. Retest and make sure you are heading in the right direction. Try retesting every 6-to-8 weeks to monitor your progress. If you are seeing progress you are on the right track. If not, then it is time to evaluate what you have been doing and try again.

Remember, if you follow this system, I promise you will see improvements in all areas of training. Trust the system and you will see improvements come.

Now let's talk about a rarely discussed topic. How you can control your recovery.

CHAPTER 3

RECOVERY

How can I do this to you? We haven't even gotten into the workouts, yet I am already discussing how you are going to recover better. It is true, we are going there. There are times you must learn how to stop before you can learn how to go.

With many of my clients, I tell them my first job is to help prevent them from getting in their own way. The concept of recovery is new to many individuals, even though it is an essential part of the program.

We tend to focus solely on pushing ourselves to the limit in our training. But you must remember allowing your body to recover is the most important part of training. If you forget this one thing you are doomed and will always get in your own way.

Your goal should not be simply to get tired in the gym. The point of a workout is not to just sweat and get sore. How sore you are is no indication of our good your workout was. The sole purpose of your training is to get better on the course. Your training is a catalyst to help your body adapt appropriately. It is ok to be sore and ok to sweat, but they are side products of your program, not the goal.

You do not get stronger or faster right after your workout. In fact, you are in worse shape than when you started. Your muscle tissue is breaking down, you have used up energy stores, and mentally you are fatigued. But this is just the stimulus that will lead to a series of reactions in your body that will get you better the next time.

But this takes time. You don't recover right away. If you are not allowing your body to recover properly, then you are always limiting your potential in each workout.

To help improve the response in training we will have different phases of training that you will go through. We will discuss this more in the training chapters.

There are things you can do to help improve recovery so you can get back to it as quickly as possible. We will divide these up into a few categories to help you get started. These include:

1.   Nutrition

2.   Sleep

3.   Soft Tissue Work

4.   Hydrotherapy

5.   Breath work

6.   Stress Management

Before we dive into each of the topics, there is an important concept I want you to understand. Your Central Nervous System (CNS) controls everything in your body. We get so caught up in building and developing muscles, but we forget what controls those muscles in the first place.

When you stress the body with exercise, or other forms of stress, the CNS will pay the price. When we focus on recovery, much of what we do is going to work towards enhancing the CNS's ability to recover. The CNS is one major factor in determining fatigue and progress. Many of the areas we touch on here will have to play a role in assisting the CNS ability to function.

For this reason, it is important to track and monitor your nervous system's status. This can be tricky to do, but technology is making this easier. For example, heart rate and heart rate variability are great ways to gain insight on your true recovery.

We have two branches of our nervous system that we will pay attention to here. This is the Parasympathetic System (Rest and Digest) and Sympathetic System (Fight or Flight). These two systems are both always active in some way. The goal is to have balance at the appropriate time. Using your heart rate we can get an idea of which system is predominantly more active at a given time.

A simple way to get started is by monitoring your heart rate every morning. You should notice it stays relatively constant. You will start to notice, however, certain times when you see an increase in your resting heart rate. This is a warning sign. A side effect of exercise should be a gradual lowering of your resting heart. This is a sign that you are on the right track. But if you notice a trend of it increasing, it is a sign of increased stress and that your body is having a harder time fully recovering.

There will be small fluctuations from day-to-day, but if you see an increase of five beats per minute or more, you will want to pay attention. I cannot back this number with hard scientific evidence, but in my experience, this is too much of an elevation. These are days that you may want to change up your plan and decrease training intensity. This doesn't mean you can't work out, but it does mean you should monitor your sessions closely.

A more sophisticated approach to monitoring is using Heart Rate Variability or HRV. This is looking at the time intervals between your heart beat. You probably know that your heart rate is not constant, like a metronome. Instead there is variability in time between each heart beat. By measuring these variations, you can estimate your recovery status by determining the influence of each of the systems of the nervous system on your heart beat. By using tools like Morpheus or HRV 4 Training you can simply take a measurement each morning that takes into count your HRV plus a few other recovery metrics, to give you a recovery baseline each day.

Now that you understand how to monitor your recovery status, let's look at a few ways to improve it.

NUTRITION

We can debate which would be more of a priority -- sleep or nutrition. Either one can be at the top of the list, but for this book's purposes we are going to start with nutrition. There is a reason the title of this book is Fuel and Fire. If you want to truly maximize your body's potential to perform its best and recover as quickly as possible you must make nutrition a priority.

It is amazing how hard people will push themselves in the gym. They crush their body repeatedly, willing to get extremely uncomfortable, yet they make little to no effort with their eating habits. If you want to see more change happen, you need to start focusing on areas you typically neglect. This is nutrition for many.

Throughout this book we will dive much deeper into nutrition and performance, but to start we will look at the healing properties of the food you eat. When you beat yourself up at the gym or deal with the daily stress of your life, your body is affected. Often, we see the body respond with inflammation. Inflammation is part of the healing process and is a naturally occurring phenomenon in the body. The problem occurs with chronic stress and inflammation. If this is left unchecked your body will never have the opportunity to adapt from the workouts you are putting yourself through.

When most people look at food they go straight to calories, wondering how they can start subtracting things from their diet. Rather, the question should be what can you add in? While calories play a role, we need to switch the emphasis to the nutrients we are putting into our body. Nutrients are the key to proper recovery, growth, and performance. We will explore the details of nutrition later in this book and learn about an anti-inflammatory diet plan.

SLEEP

Like I mentioned, we can argue whether sleep is the most important factor influencing your recovery. It is no secret that sleep is essential for optimal health and performance. But for some reason, this is often skipped over. You will see individuals purchase expensive products and supplements to try and fast-track recovery, but it is all a waste of money if you are not optimizing your sleep.

Not surprisingly, numerous studies have shown that sleep deprivation leads to decreased cognitive performance, slowed agility and quickness, decreased speed, decreased power and strength -- just to name a few.

It is not just one bad night of sleep that will land you in trouble. Instead there is something called sleep debt. Here we see that small amounts of lost sleep will start to build up into a chronic debt. And just like your student loans, this becomes a burden and must be paid back.

It is well established how bad losing sleep is, so let us focus more on what you can do about it. First, we should calculate how much sleep you need. This will be different for everyone. We can use the standard eight hours per night as a starting point. For more customized hours, the goal will be to find the amount of time needed to allow you to wake up rested and without an alarm. So, there will be some trial and error to determine this.

To improve your sleep quality, first you must answer one question. This question was suggested to me by my friend and colleague, Dr. Brandon Marcello, one of the leading experts in sleep, recovery, and performance for athletes and the military.

Here's the question: Why are you not getting the sleep you need? If you are not getting the sleep quality you need, then there must be a reason. This reason will be your priority. Answering this question will help get you closer to a better night's sleep so your body can recover from your workouts.

Are you not sleeping enough because of noise, pain, a restless partner, going to bed too late, mind racing, etc. There are many reasons why you may not be sleeping, but we must figure out the biggest contributor. Otherwise all the strategies I give you may not help.

To help get you started here are my big three for getting better sleep. These alone may be enough, but if you don't address the underlying problems first, they may not be effective.

1.   Find your schedule. You will find a consistent schedule that best fits your lifestyle. Just like most things in life, you want to develop positive habits. Your goal is to go to bed and wake up the same time each day. Yes, this means not sleeping until noon on the weekends. Keep your schedule as consistent as possible to train your body to adjust.

2.   Keep a journal by your bed. One of the common complaints I hear about lack of sleep is it is hard to turn off your thoughts. For example, you may find yourself ruminating about work as you struggle to fall asleep. This can be a very big challenge but doing a brain dump may help. If you have ideas, to do lists, or any other thoughts in your head, get them out by writing them

all down. It is a signal to your brain that you acknowledge the thoughts and you will deal with them at a later time when you can focus.

3. Keep it cooler. Our body operates off circadian rhythms. We have all probably heard that our bodies, normally, will follow a 24-hour sleep/wake cycle. Similarly, we have a core temperature cycle that follows the same pattern. We see our core temperature drop during nocturnal activities and rise during daytime activities. Warm environments have been shown to disrupt different phases of sleep. So, keep your room on the cooler side to help follow these patterns. The best temperature seems to be between 60-67 degrees Fahrenheit.

SOFT-TISSUE WORK

There is something special about having a foam roller get to know every inch of your body. Improved movement should always be the goal. Move better and you will perform better. Move better and you will live better. Mobility restrictions are just all too common these days and while foam rolling will not address all these restrictions, it is a good place to start. Besides, we will need every advantage we can get in order to improve movement and tissue health.

It is still not perfectly clear what foam rolling or other soft tissue work does. Having hands-on work from a massage therapist or other soft-tissue professional is always the best option. But let's be more practical and focus on using a foam roller or other tool that can be used to work your muscles on your own.

When talking about foam rolling you may often hear the term self-myofascial release. Whether you are releasing fascia during foam rolling is not clear -- and most likely not the case. But it does work. It helps with trigger points, inflammation, active release, and increased body awareness. Many research papers have shown that foam rolling improves range of motion without decreases in performance measures. This is exactly what we are looking for.

We will get into the specifics on what, how, and when to foam roll as we get into your programming, but just understand that this is an essential, non-negotiable part of training. If you don't have a foam roller, buy one right now.

HYDROTHERAPY

There is something special about being in water. We will discuss hot and cold therapy, but just the act of being suspended in water is a powerful recovery tool for your body. Think of all the stress you put your muscles and joints through during a typical day. When you get in water you start to take body weight off. This reduction is a great way to stimulate recovery and healing.

One research study showed that water immersion at a temperature of 32 degrees Celsius can reduce heart rate by 15% and blood pressure by 11%. A decrease in levels of plasma cortisol -- a stress hormone -- was also registered. Hydrotherapy has even been shown to boost the immune system.

Cold water immersion has shown similar effects. And when you combine hot and cold therapy (known as contrast therapy) you can receive additional benefits. Six minutes of alternating between one minute hot and one minute cold has been shown to reduce muscle soreness, pain, and stiffness.

The hardest part about these methods are often logistics. But running a hot bath and then jumping back and forth between a cold shower and hot bath is a simple way to apply contrast therapy in your home.

BREATH WORK

It is amazing how we look straight to the most advanced and complicated technologies and techniques for training, when the most effective tool is usually the simplest thing you can do.

Breathing is one of those things. We do not have to belabor the point of how important breathing is. Try holding your breath for as long as you can. Most likely the sensors in your body will prevent you from really doing any damage, sending you very strong signals for you to breathe. Even if you are tough enough to ignore these signs, you will eventually pass out, and your brain will take over so you cannot do any permanent damage.

The two big pieces I want to bring up for breathing -- pieces that will provide you with immediate recovery benefits -- are the roles it plays within nervous system activity and mobility. While we need to get oxygen in and carbon dioxide out in order to live, for our purposes with recovery we will focus on these two areas.

To keep things brief, our autonomic nervous system is broken into two branches; sympathetic and parasympathetic, as mentioned previously. Both branches are critical for performance; one, to handle the stress thrown at us during everyday life and training bouts; and the other to help improve recovery and absorption of nutrients we take in.

Most people forget about the importance of the nervous system. While a muscle must recover after a workout, if the nervous system isn't ready for another tough session, there will be a reduction in performance. This is a result of how the nervous system controls everything. So, if the nervous system isn't working right, nothing else will. When we constantly stress our bodies -- and yes, exercise is stress -- we see a shift to sympathetic dominant activity. Elevated sympathetic activity over prolonged periods of time is a recipe for overtraining, injury, and decreased performance.

Breathing is a simple and effective way for enhancing parasympathetic activity. Plus, you are taking time to relax and focus on your body, which are always great things to do. Simply by focusing on breathing you can have direct interaction with your nervous system.

So breathing practice helps create a better environment for recovery. Additional benefits from the increased parasympathetic activity are core stability and joint mobility improvements.

How can simply breathing do all of this? Well, first, when you focus on better quality breathing, you are elevating the ability of the diaphragm to do its job. The diaphragm's first job is to assist with breathing. It also creates initial core stability. Without this deep core stability, we are more likely to develop compensations.

Improper breathing patterns are responsible for compensations that lead to decreased mobility, poor posture, and increased risk of injury. Yes, all of these issues can arise simply by not breathing right. When the diaphragm isn't working properly, other muscles will pick up the slack. For example, muscles of the neck and shoulder start to assist more with breathing, meaning they are engaged all the time. This will cause them to be tight and restricted. You would be amazed how much better your neck and shoulders feel after a few simple breathing drills.

Considering all the major benefits you receive from breathing exercises, this is just something you must include on a regular basis. So, of course you are already breathing each day. But our goal is to achieve better quality breaths. To find out if you have a breathing dysfunction you can start with two simple assessments.

First, take a normal inhalation; then exhale. After a normal exhale, plug your nose, and hold your breath. Do not hold it as long as you possibly can. Instead, time how long you can hold your breath until you feel the first significant urge to breathe. Then stop the timer. If you cannot hold this for 30 seconds, there is a good possibility you have a breathing issue.

Next you will perform a max hold on the inhalation. For this test you will push to see how long you can hold your breath after a normal inhale. This duration should be at least 60 seconds. If you fall short on either or both assessments, then there is a good chance you will benefit from some direct breath work.

I want to leave you with two easy drills to start with. These are crocodile breathing and cat camel breathing. For the crocodile breathing exercise, you will lie face down on the floor with your hands under your forehead. It is important to stay relaxed throughout the drill. Next you will inhale through your nose. As you inhale your diaphragm is contracting. The diaphragm muscle is a 360 degree dome that will push out on all sides of the trunk. You will feel your belly push into the floor. As this happens your lower back should rise up. Hold the inhale for a second or two. Then exhale completely, feeling your lower back drop back down and hold the end of the exhale for a few seconds. Repeat this drill for one to two minutes.

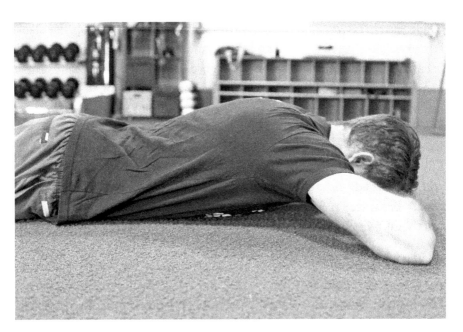

Crocodile Breathing

With the cat camel breathing, you probably have seen and already done this exercise, but now we will be more intentional with our breathing. You will associate extension, or the cat portion, with inhalation and flexion, the camel portion, with exhalation. When you take your spine through full extension you will take a deep inhalation and hold for two to three seconds. Then exhale and go through full exhalation and again hold for two or three seconds.

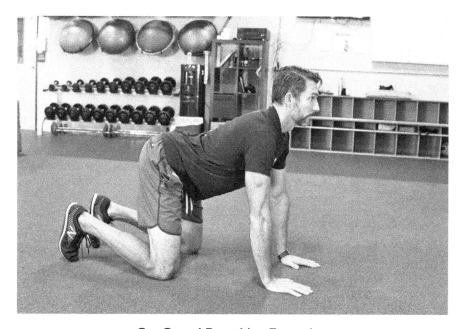

Cat Camel Breathing Extension

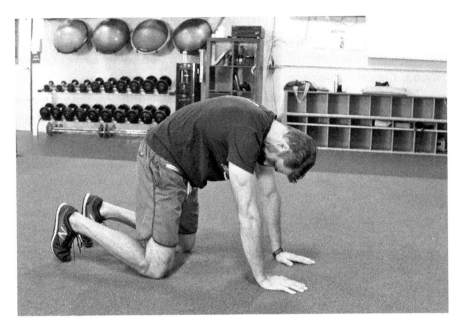

Cat Camel Breathing Flexion

STRESS MANAGEMENT

In this short section I will show you how to remove all stress from your life. I wish...

There are different directions we can focus on stress management and, honestly, full books have been written on each of them. For our purposes, I want you to be aware of the stress that is being placed on your body and not eliminate it but manage it.

Now, we have already discussed the nervous systems role in recovery. The goal should be to have a balance between parasympathetic and sympathetic activity. If we are constantly training hard, there will be a shift to more sympathetic activity. This opens us up to more inflammation, injury, illness, burnout, and other issues. As we discussed, breath work is a great way to help improve this balance and speed up recovery. Many enjoy meditation, being outdoors, or other ways to deal with stress.

It is critical that we understand when we are under too much stress. Sometimes it is obvious with how you feel. You just know when you did too much. But this is a very reactive approach and it is now too late. You have no choice but to back off and wait until you are ready to go again.

I have already discussed using heart rate and heart rate variability as tools to help determine when you are overly stressed. This should not be used just for exercise. When you have other stressors in your life, these numbers will reflect it. Keep an eye so you know when to back off and focus extra attention on your recovery.

The last piece of advice I can give on managing stress is realizing you only have control over your reaction to things. This is a stoic philosophy that you can read more on in books like Ryan Holliday's The Obstacle Is The Way, or Letters From A Stoic by Seneca. These will hopefully shed some light on how to deal with things that don't go your way.

All of the aspects of recovery that we have discussed so far are easy to do. They will go a long way in preparing you for your training to maximize the adaptations that your body should be going through from all your hard work.

Now let's get into the training side.

CHAPTER 4

ENDURANCE

Now that our body is primed for the stresses that will be placed on it with workouts, it is time to start looking at our first exercise section: endurance. It wasn't until I fully embraced the idea of endurance training that I saw major breakthroughs in my own training.

OCR's are typically longer events that require us to maximize our body's capability to endure large stresses. It seems simple enough to assume to go out and run for a long period of time and your endurance will just improve. This, however, isn't always going to be the best path. You need to look at how your body's physiology works to understand how you can effectively train and maximize your results. When you fully understand the concepts that will be brought up in this chapter, you are going to see massive breakthroughs in your training and your race day performance. The key areas to focus on are energy systems and your body's ability to use fuel efficiently. If you can figure out how to do this, you're going to improve leaps and bounds in your performance.

A unique aspect of this book is that we are going to be breaking down not only the training but the fueling behind the training. When you understand how your body produces and uses energy, you'll better understand how to eat right to match your training. This is the path toward optimal results. In this first section we are going to look at how your body creates energy from carbohydrates and fats. Yes, it may help to have a degree in exercise physiology, but I don't believe it is necessary to understand how this works.

ENERGY SYSTEMS: THE BASICS

When you have an understanding of how the body supplies energy to the muscles in order to do work, you will have the knowledge of types of food to eat and types of training to incorporate. If you want a deeper dive into energy systems, you can pick up an Exercise Physiology textbook. But to save you some time, I will go over the basics that you should know.

There are three systems that we use for energy. The first system is the Creatine Phosphagen System. This system is great for providing the immediate energy needed for running a short sprint, jumping over a wall, or picking up a heavy weight. The problem is we can only use this energy system for a few seconds before it can't support the exercise. This system will primarily rely on stored energy in the muscle tissue.

The next system is called the Glycolytic System. Here you are now breaking down carbohydrates, glucose and glycogen, to produce fuel. This system begins to take over when the Creatine Phosphagen System can no longer support the exercise. The Glycolytic System can produce energy without the presence of oxygen, making it fast to kick in, but like our first system, it can only support high intensity exercise for a relatively short period of time. In the case of the Glycolytic System, this equals a few minutes. After this, you'll depend on the final system to continue supporting your effort.

Our last system is the Oxidative System. Here we are burning fats or further breaking down carbs for more energy. Since we need oxygen present for this system to work, it takes a few minutes before it can kick in to support exercise. For long duration exercise, the Oxidative

System is what we use to fuel from a few minutes of movement to hours of movement.

It's important to note that there is no one system completely supporting our efforts. They all work together, but at different degrees. For example, you may be running at a slower pace during a race, using the Oxidative System primarily to support the effort. But then you have to run and jump over a few walls in the middle of this run. In these moments you will need help from the Glycolytic System in order for this to happen.

YOUR GOAL IN TRAINING

Your goal in training will be to become as efficient as possible within each of these systems. This is referred to as energy systems development. In order to do this you need to spend time training in each system with deliberation. Many will try and push as hard as they can as long as they can. While sometimes this is an effective workout, it cannot be the entire plan.

When you understand how these systems operate, you will know what types of food you should be consuming to fuel each workout. We will cover the nutrition later in this book. For now we will focus on how to train in each system.

As we examine typical OCR events, they will be composed of varying distances starting at a few miles and extending to the marathon distance, or more. Each type of race will have a specific training plan to support the energy systems needed for the race. Whichever type of race you will be running, your goal is to optimize each of these different energy systems. You just may spend more or less time in certain ones depending on the distance.

As mentioned, all race distances will require using all three energy systems. In races where very short distances are covered (and typically with more lifting), such as an Epic Series, you will be calling on the first energy system greatly, with support from the anaerobic system. In shorter running races -- as in under 5 miles -- you will need much more help from the anaerobic system with additional support from the aerobic or Oxidative System. Races of longer distances will heavily rely on the aerobic system, but don't forget the help from the anaerobic systems.

UPGRADE YOUR TRAINING

With an understanding of how the energy systems work, it is now time to find how you can use this knowledge to inform smarter training. The main idea is that you will spend time in each of the different systems or training zones. There are a few different ways to do this, but we will start with a three-zone system for simplicity.

Think of these training zones as low intensity, moderate intensity, and high intensity. The problem that most people run into is they try and push hard all the time. But really you can't push hard for that long. So, what happens? Many athletes gett stuck in the moderate-intensity zone. In the distance running world this is often described as junk mileage. The problem with spending all of your time here is you never are truly training aerobically or anaerobically with much efficiency. This means neither will be maximized. You will still see improvements, but they will be significantly limited.

To unlock your full potential, you will follow a program that strategically trains different zones. Each zone is dependent on your physiology. You can perform laboratory testing, such as VO2 max testing, to get incredibly accurate heart rates at certain physiological markers. But we will use more practical testing to determine your specific heart rate parameters.

CHART YOUR ZONES

To chart your heart rate zones you will first need to determine your maximum aerobic threshold and lactate threshold. Your maximum aerobic threshold is the highest intensity where you can support exercise with the aerobic or oxidative system. At this point you are primarily using fats for fuel. As you raise intensity from this point, you will start increasing your needs from the anaerobic systems and carbohydrates.

As you increase the demand on the anaerobic systems, you are breaking down more and more sugar through glycolysis. A byproduct of this process is lactate. Lactate initially is not a big deal. It will flow into your bloodstream and then be transported to the liver. There it is converted to glucose for more energy. The problem is you can only do this for so long before lactate builds up in the blood. This buildup will eventually cause fatigue in the muscle and interfere with performance.

Your lactate threshold is the point when this happens. When you hit this intensity, you will typically only be able to maintain it for around 30 minutes.

With training you can improve both your aerobic and lactate threshold. When you train the right way, both points will occur at higher intensities. This means you can run at faster paces at each. You now understand the importance of knowing about producing energy to support training so now let's get into your numbers.

AEROBIC TRAINING ZONE

For the maximum aerobic training zone we can use a formula created by the great running coach Phil Maffetone. You simply use the formula 180 – your age in order to get a starting point for your numbers. Use the chart below for any necessary adjustments.

Phil Maffetone's 180 Formula
1. Subtract your age from 180.
2. Adjust the number based on the following categories:

	* If you have or are recovering from a major illness or are on any regular medication, subtract an additional 10.
	* If you are injured, have regressed in training or competition, get more than two colds or bouts of flu per year, have allergies or asthma, or if you have been inconsistent or are just getting back into training, subtract an additional 5.
	* If you have been training consistently (at least four times per week) for up to two years without any of the problems mentioned above keep the number the same.
	* If you have been training for more than two years without any of the problems above, and have made progress in competition without injury, add 5.

LACTATE THRESHOLD

For your lactate threshold, please revisit Chapter 2 and your assessment of cardiorespiratory endurance. This is the number we will use for your point of high intensity. You now can fill in your numbers for your training zones.

- Zone 1 will include any training performed at an intensity at or below your aerobic threshold.
- Zone 2 will be anything between your aerobic and lactate threshold.
- Zone 3 is anything above your lactate threshold. Since we will be using heart rates at each of these points, if you do not currently have a heart rate monitor, I strongly recommend it.

Next, we will look at the specific training you can do for each of these zones.

CHAPTER 5

CARDIORESPIRATORY WORKOUTS

When you look at much of the research evaluating elite runners, you will see an interesting phenomenon. They spend most of their training in Zone 1, or lower intensity training. This goes against what many are currently doing. It is easy to assume that more is better, and that intensity should be pushed as much as possible. But in reality, the opposite seems to be the most effective.

For example, we can look at research from the Journal of Strength and Conditioning Research. Scientists compared the effects on performance in a 10km run between subjects who spent 80% of their time training in Zone 1 versus subjects who spent 65% of their time in Zone 1. In this study they matched their Zone 3 training at 10% so the main difference was Zone 2 training.

The good news is that both groups saw improvements in their 10k times. So, both seem to be effective for training, but we are not only looking for effectiveness. Your goal should be to maximize your results. And in this study the group that trained more in Zone 1 saw an average improvement of 7% versus only 1.6% in the other group. Over 5% improvements and you work out at lower intensity? Sign me up.

Now, it is worth bringing up that the studies supporting this approach are solely focused on running, cycling, and other traditional endurance events; not OCRs. But we can still learn from this. Depending on the race, you might spend more or less time in each zone.

PURPOSE BEHIND EACH WORKOUT

The big lesson to take from this concept is to have a specific purpose behind each workout you do. If you can take away this one point, you will be miles ahead of the majority of racers. You really can't have it all in each workout and there is no such thing as the perfect workout. You will choose what you need and focus on that area.

For example, if your running workouts primarily consist of running as hard as you can for as long as you can go, you are significantly limiting your potential. Previously, I brought up the idea of junk or garbage miles. There is much literature already written on this topic, and one that I have extensively covered on my podcast. But it is worth mentioning.

The term 'junk miles' refers to training performed in that no man's land. Remember the goal of training is to stress your body and the different physiological systems within, in order to adapt so you become more efficient. With OCR training we are trying to focus on improving both anaerobic systems of energy production and aerobic systems. By lowering intensity you are stressing your aerobic system more efficiently, hence you will see bigger improvement in aerobic metabolism and fat utilization. Higher intensity training improves anaerobic systems and better carbohydrate utilization.

When you train both systems effectively you will develop better metabolic flexibility, meaning you can switch between different fuel sources much more effectively. This leads to better overall performance and less likelihood of bonking during a race. Metabolic flexibility is a key concept we will discuss later in this book.

When you are training at a pace that is hard but not as hard as you can go, you get stuck between these two places. So you really aren't maximizing aerobic or anaerobic systems appropriately. This is what we mean by junk miles.

Now that this is clear we can look at the specific training you can do in each zone. There may be some workouts that are in that middle zone, but this is by design and not performed all the time.

As we review each workout you will perform, there will be some that include training in all three zones. These workouts will be categorized by which zone they are intended to spend the most time improving. There are times when you will try and push your lactate threshold -- and these workouts will help. The main point is do not perform all of your workouts in the lactate threshold zone.

ZONE 1 WORKOUTS

With Zone 1 workouts, we are referring to any workouts that are just at or below your maximum aerobic threshold heart rate. So really any activity that keeps your heart rate under that intensity will do. This includes non-structured activities. For our structured running or cross training plan we will include three primary workouts.

Long Slow Distance Runs

The drug, LSD, may not help much with endurance training, but LSD (long slow distance) workouts are a great fit. These workouts are essentially designed to add more miles to your training. The primary focus of these workouts is to hit a certain mileage goal and improve your aerobic threshold.

How far you will be running will be determined by the phase of training and the specific race you will be training for. While any race distance will have some form of LSD training, you will be looking to focus on this type of workout for longer races of 8 or more miles. As a rule I usually work backwards from race day. First you determine what your longest run distance will be. This distance you will probably hit anywhere from 2-4 weeks before your race, depending on the distance. Then you can subtract 10% every 1-2 weeks to have a nice progression for race day.

This can be challenging for those who like to push the pace. Try and make the goal distance covered, rather than pace. You will only run as fast as you can while staying under your aerobic threshold. So set your ego aside here and focus on quality of the miles versus pure speed. Don't worry, we will get to speed later.

FOUNDATION RUNS

Foundation runs will be similar to LSD runs with one key difference. Instead of focusing on distance, you will focus on time. This is where you will likely log most of your weekly miles. Foundation runs will typically range from 30-to-90 minutes of continuous lower-intensity running. But remember, you will stay within the aerobic zone of training so keep the intensity lower here.

RECOVERY RUNS

Your final Zone 1 runs will be for recovery. These will be the lowest intensity runs. You will want to stay at a pace below your aerobic threshold here. This would be that 'forever' pace. Once you settle in you could stay here for a long time.

To help get an idea of what this pace should be, I usually recommend nasal breathing only. If you have to breathe through your mouth during a recovery run, you are pushing too hard.

Zone 1 workouts, like foundation runs, will be based on time, ranging from 30-to-60 minutes. The goal is just to move. These work well on days that you are sore and need more time to recover but still want to get in a workout, after a race when you aren't quite ready to get back into it yet, or even for a taper before a race.

So, remember the focus is remaining in an aerobic heart rate zone for these sessions, so keep an eye on your heart rate monitor to remain in check. The longer the race distance the more Zone 1 workouts you will find yourself doing.

ZONE 2 WORKOUTS

As you have previously read, Zone 2 refers to workouts that put you in the intensity between your aerobic capacity and your lactate threshold. This area is not a perfect fit for aerobic or anaerobic training.

I want to make it clear that this type of training is not bad; it just gets often overused. When you aren't applying it properly with adequate Zone 1 and Zone 3 training, you run the risk of limiting your performance.

Many races that you will be performing will be at this type of intensity, so it is important you still train in Zone 2. Just don't make this the only type of training you are doing in your running and cross training.

Zone 2 training will help improve your lactate threshold, which means you can work at higher intensities before hitting this marker. You get better at clearing lactate from your blood so you can push these higher intensities for longer. This is the perfect recipe for a faster race pace.

TEMPO RUNS

You may have heard tempo runs referred to as race-pace training. I suggest using these terms interchangeably. The idea here is you are running at your typical race pace. This will vary depending on the distance you are racing -- and since you will be hitting obstacles during a race -- you can't employ normal OCR race pace.

Instead, you will focus on the fastest pace you can sustain for the given time or distance you will be running. I personally like to use time for these workouts. After a 5-to-10 minute warm up you will perform the fastest pace you can for 10-40 minutes.

Since these are workouts at your lactate threshold, you likely won't be able to maintain this intensity for more than 40 minutes. If you can, then you are an exception. More commonly, you're not running hard enough during the workout.

FAST FINISH RUNS

Fast finish runs are just what they sound like. It is essentially a foundation run or LSD run with a tempo run added to the end. So, this is a combination of Zone 1 and 2. The first part of the workout will be a lower intensity aerobic run. This can be a timedbased run or measured in miles. Then you will finish as fast as you can for a set time or distance. This is one of my favorite Zone 2-type workouts to perform.

The idea with fast finish runs is to improve metabolic efficiency as you improve the aerobic and anaerobic systems. When you start the run, if you are fueling and training properly, you will primarily be using fat for fuel. This is great because you will supply more energy that will last longer. But at the end of a race you need to have some fuel in the tank to sprint to the finish. This will come from carbohydrates and the anaerobic system.

The fast finish run is a great way to train for this. You start aerobically then finish fast anaerobically. An example could be:

5 Minute Warm up
25 Minute Foundation Run
10 Minute Fast Finish

Or if you are using mileage:

1 Mile Warm up
6 Mile LSD Run
1 Mile Fast Finish

CAPACITY INTERVALS

There are many different forms of interval training workouts you will see. Most people are familiar with High Intensity Interval Training. This involves short, very intense bursts of exercise followed by an active or passive recovery.

Depending on how intense and how long your intervals are it will train your cardiorespiratory system differently. With capacity intervals we are performing moderate intensity intervals but for longer periods of time. Even though I am using the term moderate, these are still challenging.

The goal here is to improve your anaerobic capacity. These can be performed on hills or flat surfaces. The length of the work period will be in the range of 2-to-5 minutes. Your intensity will be running as hard as you can for that amount of time.

These fall within Zone 2 intensity because they are longer intervals, and by definition you won't be able to maintain a pace or heart rate high enough to be considered Zone 3. But it will be close.

Your recovery periods will vary depending on your level of fitness. In my experience, if you are using a heart-rate monitor, you can begin your next interval when you hit 65-to-70% of your max heart rate. I prefer using heart rate for recovery, but if you use time you will likely start with a 1:2 work-to-rest ratio. You may potentially shorten your recovery to about a 1:.5 work-to-rest ratio.

FARTLEK OR SPEEDPLAY

Fartlek is the funny Swedish word meaning speed play. This is essentially just an interval workout, but we typically don't see the same structured work-to-rest ratio. Because of this, it becomes difficult to program these types of workouts.

The two simplest ways to structure Fartlek training is with time or distance. For the former you will set a period of running time ranging anywhere from 30-to-90 minutes. Within this time frame you will perform random bursts of moderate-intensity intervals.

Imagine running with a friend and seeing a building at the end of the road. You turn to your friend and say, "race you to the building!" Then the two of you burst into a sprint to get there. Once you arrive you slow down and continue to run a slower pace again. Then your friend challenges you to a race at another spot during the run. You continue this game throughout the session.

If you need more structure you might follow a program based on how many miles you want to run. Let's say you want to run for eight miles. After your warm up, you run the first ¼ mile at a harder pace, then back off to a slower pace for the rest of the mile. You perform 8 rounds of this for your 8 mile run.

ZONE 3 WORKOUTS

Your final category of workouts will be your highest intensity training. For these to truly be Zone 3-type workouts, you must be hitting sufficient intensities. Many athletes not ready or willing to perform this kind of exercise. Make sure you build up to this.

The intensity in Zone 3 must be above your lactate threshold. You cannot train at this intensity for very long, so it has to be broken up with intervals. The max amount of time for each interval should not exceed

90 seconds; and even this is for highly-trained individuals. Realistically, most will be sticking with 10-to-60 seconds for their sprints.

In Zone 3, your recovery should be much longer than your work period. You want each sprint to be all-out, so if you are not recovering enough between each interval, you won't achieve the necessary intensity or maintain a fast enough pace throughout the workout.

Use your heart rate for recovery, See how resting until you slow to 65% of your max heart rate works for you. But most crucial, pay attention to your pacing for each sprint. If you are not hitting what you should be, you will want to increase your rest period. Using timed recovery, you will likely be using a 1:3-to-6 work-to-rest ratio.

During your rest, it is best to perform an active recovery. This means you will be moving in some way during your rest versus just standing or sitting down. A simple walk is enough here, but more conditioned athletes may even jog between sprints. I cannot stress enough the importance of adequate recovery to maintain your goal pace during each sprint.

Just like the capacity intervals, this can be performed on flat or hills. It is probably best to mix it up and do both.

A GREAT STARTING POINT

These examples do not comprise all the running workouts for each zone, but it is a good start for you to play with. You will not be performing every workout each week. In fact, sometimes you are not going to hit every zone each week. This is where periodization, planning, and program design come into place.

A great starting point is, at the minimum, log one workout from each zone each week. However, based on the race distance you are training for you may tweak this some. For example, if you are running a shorter race, as in less than 5 miles, you will spend more time in zones 2 and 3. If you are training for a 15 miles-or-more race you will be focusing much of your training in the Zone 1 workouts.

You won't exclude any zone in preparing for any type of race, just adjust the numbers to best reflect what you will see in the specific race you are targeting. If you aren't sure if you are doing it right, there is always trial and error. If you measured your cardiorespiratory fitness using one of the mentioned assessments, you can retest to make sure you are registering progress.

If all of this seems overwhelming, don't worry. You will be able to see what a sample plan looks like using these workouts as our foundation.

I intentionally discussed your running program first and how you can improve your energy systems, because I believe it is usually the most lacking piece of most OCR training programs. Remember these are races and you need to run. If you are too worn out by the time you get to the obstacle you won't have a chance anyway.

That said, many runners make the big mistake of excluding strength workouts from their program. This is a mistake you will not make. In the next chapter I will share everything you need to build a result-driven strength program.

CHAPTER 6

STRENGTH TRAINING

I have always been biased toward strength training. This is what I grew up doing and fell in love with. Getting stronger has so many real-life applications. Clearly it will turn you into a better racer.

But the idea that you can just pick up heavy weights and automatically see an improvement is a mistake. As mentioned, if you want to get stronger and more powerful, you first must move well. Only then will you have positive adaptations to your training sessions. If you haven't evaluated your movement by a professional or through a self-screen, get it done.

When you do move well, strength training has numerous benefits. There is the obvious that you will be stronger and more powerful, increasing your chances of completing obstacles, but maybe more importantly, it will improve your running economy (aka efficiency)and reduce your risk of injury.

Strength training has been shown to strengthen not only muscles, but bone, connective tissue, and joints. This will help you stay more durable with all the impact stress that comes with training and racing. Strength training can improve your running economy, which means you will be more efficient during your runs. When you are more efficient, you use less energy and will not need to work as hard. This means you will be able to maintain faster paces for longer.

Another big benefit of strength training is it lowers your perceived exertion. Perceived exertion refers to how hard you feel you are pushing during a workout. So not only will you be able to run faster for longer, but it won't feel as hard as it previously did.

Hopefully, I don't need to sell strength training to you and you're ready to go. You may be somewhat familiar with strength training, but I want to make sure we go over all the aspects of training you should consider. This includes the components of a strength workout plus periodization or different progressions to follow. Then I want to leave you with a few baselines to see if you are strong enough or need to make more improvements.

COMPONENTS OF A STRENGTH WORKOUT

It helps sometimes to think of your workout as steps or checkpoints. You will want to make sure you check the box for as many items as you can. Sometimes you may not be able to train for everything, but if you know what you missed in one workout, you can make up for it in another one.

Here I want to review the different components for your workout. You will want to check off as many of these components as you can. But every person will be different. Some will need more work in one area and less in another. Therefore, knowing your strengths and weaknesses will be important.

MOVEMENT PREPARATION

Yes, this is a fancy word for your warm-up. But really "warm-up" is such a bad term to describe what you are trying to do. Sure, one portion of this section is intended to increase your core temperature to prepare for the workout, but this will happen as a result of all the other exercises you will perform so we do not need to stress upon it.

Instead, think of this as time to prepare your body for what you need to do. You will want to know your common issues here and really try and work on them. I can spend an entire book on this section, but I will stick to the main points for you to get started with.

Before we get too far into the exercises, there is an important concept I want you to understand. It involves how the joints of the body work together through a balance of stability and mobility to create efficient movement. When this balance is thrown off, we see dysfunctional movement patterns, which lead to overuse and injury. When this occurs, you can't race or train as much as you would like to.

This joint by joint approach of stability and mobility is incredibly important. The concept first came to the fitness world from world renown experts, Mike Boyle and Gray Cook. These names may not mean much to you, but in the fitness and performance worlds, these are two very influential people.

To simplify this concept, each joint of the body has one of two primary roles. The joint is designed for stability or mobility. Now all joints need to be stable and mobile, but this concept is looking at the joints main role during functional movement.

To cover the main joints, we can start at the ankle and see how mobile this joint should be. The ankle needs to move in three planes of motion. Then we can move to the knee and see that while the knee should move, it needs to remain stable during movement. Picture someone squatting and seeing the knees come together. This would be an example of an unstable joint.

If you continue up the chain to the hips, again we find a very mobile joint. Next up is the lumbar spine, designed for stability. The thoracic spine, our next joint, is designed for significantly more mobility. The scapulo-thoracic joint is needed for stability. Then the glenohumeral, or shoulder joint, is needed to be very mobile.

These are just some of the main joints, but we see this alternating role of stability and mobility throughout the body. We need this balance to create more efficient movement and keep our joints functioning properly to maximize performance and reduce wear and tear.

For many individuals we see a switch in roles. For example, if you lack the appropriate ankle mobility, you will often see a compensation expressed within another joint, like the knee. This might be where the knees cave in during a squat, because the ankle cannot support the movement properly.

Or maybe you lack adequate hip mobility and your lumbar spine makes up the difference. So every time you bend down to pick something up you will compensate with excessive lumbar spine movement.

So why are we even talking about this? If you have a better understanding of which joints of the body need maximal movement and which need more work on stability, it helps us design a better warm up routine to prepare for the stress we are about to put your body under.

With this knowledge we can examine all of the different areas of focus for the movement preparation phase of the workout. This includes mobility which will involve soft tissue work and stretching exercises, stability exercise, and corrective drills. Many of these exercises overlap, but for our explanation we can separate them.

To give you a few ideas of how to prepare for each workout we will go through a few examples of each. Every person is different and will benefit from different exercises. The goal isn't necessarily to go through all of these, every workout, but keep them in mind in regards to areas of weakness that could use the most attention.

BREATH WORK

We have already discussed breathing in the recovery section of this book. It is worth bringing up again. For many, breath work is a great start to a workout. If improper breathing patterns are occurring, then often the muscles of the neck and shoulders are overactive.

When this occurs, it will limit mobility and increase tension in the neck and shoulders. Also, when we redevelop better diaphragmatic breathing patterns, we can establish better core and lumbar stability.

A perfect place to start is with the breathing exercises mentioned earlier, such as crocodile breathing and cat cow breathing. But remember, good breathing can be part of any exercise, so we are always working on breath.

SOFT-TISSUE WORK

Now that you are relaxed and in a good position from your breathing, we can start with soft tissue work. This typically means self-myofascial release using a foam roller, massage stick, lacrosse ball, or other self-myofascial tool.

We will break the specific exercises up and match them to the joint they are designed to improve mobility for.

There are a few important concepts to consider when rolling. Use these as guidelines to get the most out of it.

MAKE ROLLING EFFECTIVE

Work the entire muscle. You may have certain "hot spots" or trigger points in areas, but make sure you include the entire muscle.

Less is more. You only need to exert a few pounds of pressure when rolling. Despite what many believe, you don't have to crush your muscles. If you are in so much pain that you are holding your breath and turning red, you are creating too much pressure.

Form a mental picture. It may be uncomfortable but try and picture your muscle melting around the roller or object you are working with. Remember we are trying to relax and loosen the tissue, not tighten it back up.

Focus on the goal then move on. There is no strict time you should be spending on each area. In fact, you may find yourself rolling longer on certain areas than others as well. The goal is that the muscle feels better than when you started. Once you have hit that point you can probably move on. We don't want you spending 30 minutes sitting on a foam roller. Roll the muscles then move on.

Here are some of the essential rolling targets you can get started with. Please note that you can find videos of all of the exercises listed in this book at www.ocrunderground.com/book-bonus

The Ankle

1. Plantar Fascia

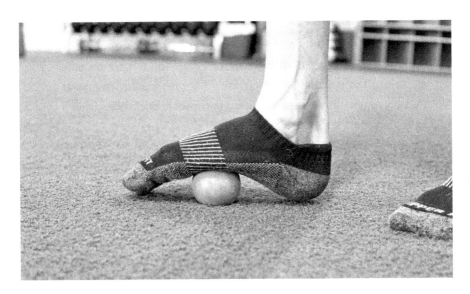

2. Calves

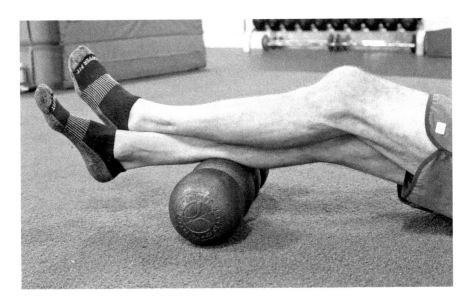

3. Anterior Tibialis

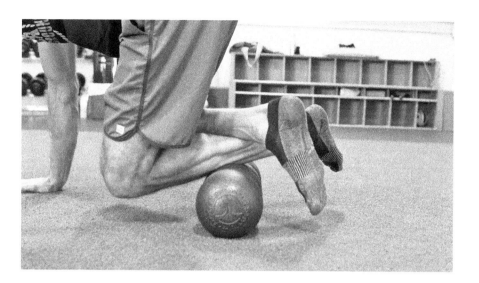

The Hips

4. Quadriceps

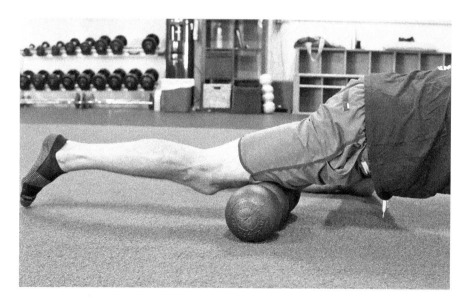

5. Adductors

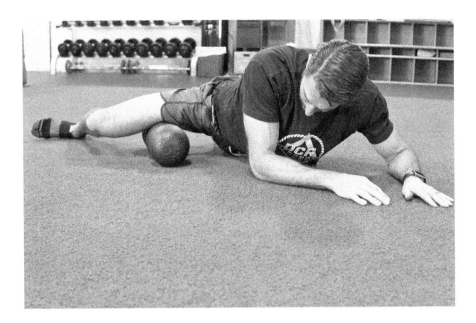

6. Hip Rotators

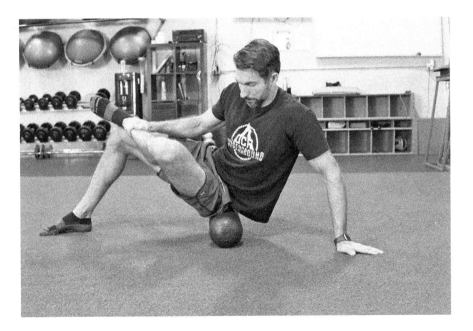

The Shoulders and Thoracic Spine

7. T-spine

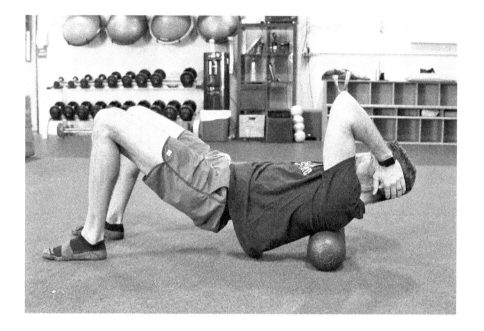

8. Pectorals

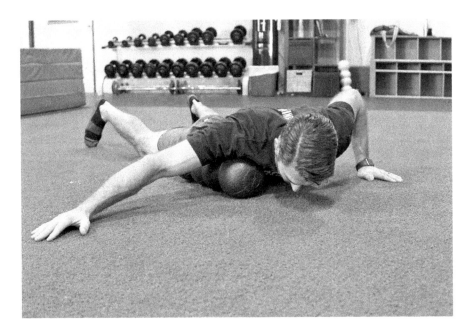

9. Latissimus Dorsi

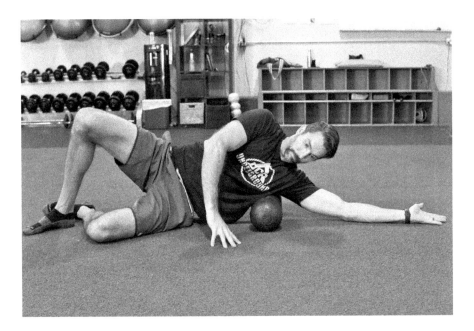

10. Triceps

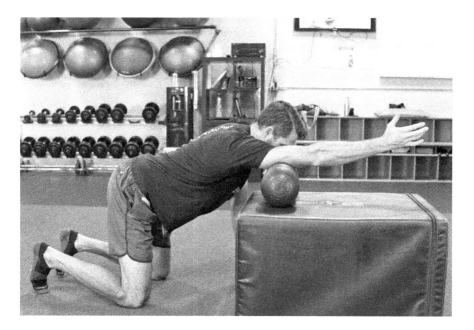

STRETCHING

Stretching can be a very hot topic. Now that you have improved tissue quality and reduced the density of muscle, it is time to lengthen the tissue to improve range of motion around a joint. There are many different forms of stretching you can do. They all have their benefits.

One issue I want to bring up involves static stretching before training. This is the type of stretching that involves lengthening a muscle and holding a position of a stretch for a prolonged period of time. This has been a debated topic for quite some time. Many believe that stretching a muscle reduces the power a muscle can produce and should never be done before exercise.

While there is some truth to that, it is more important to remember the role of stretching and the priorities of each individual. If you are extremely limited in your range of motion, and get positive outcomes from static stretching, you may want to do it before training.

It is not like you kill a muscle when you stretch it. It just temporarily loses capacity to express max power production. For many this isn't a big issue. But either way, you won't want to statically stretch and then go right into your lifting or other training. You will do things as part of your warm-up to help restore that power before your big lifts.

Along with static stretching, dynamic stretching and proprioceptive neuromuscular facilitation stretching (aka PNF), will be useful techniques. As we did with the foam rolling exercises above you will find a few essentials below that will help improve mobility for the ankle, hip, thoracic spine, and shoulder.

You most likely will not perform all of these. Test a few out to see what areas work the best for you. As mentioned with foam rolling, don't forget to breathe. This is a great spot for breathwork. We want these stretches to hold after you perform them. If you are pushing too hard into a stretch or holding your breath, your body will view this as a painful position. The body is always going to do its best to avoid pain.

To get the most out of your stretching you can follow these guidelines for each stretch.

STRETCHING BASICS

Static stretching

Complete full breaths in each position. Inhale deeply and hold for 2 seconds then exhale complete and hold for 2 seconds. Instead of timing the position, hold for 5-8 breaths. As long as you can complete full breaths you are probably in a deep enough stretch.

Dynamic Stretching

Complete full range of motion with every rep. Each rep see if you can get just a bit further. Work your breath in with each rep.

PNF

Continue to work on good breathing patterns. There will be more descriptions below with specific exercises, but hold isometric contractions for 10-20 seconds in each position. Then try and move deeper into each stretch with each rep.

Specific Stretches

Many of the stretches below will involve different areas and patterns within the body, so you will find certain stretches don't only stretch the area listed.

Remember, you can find videos of all exercises listed in this book at www.ocrunderground.com/book-bonus

Ankle Mobilization

1. Toe Sitting Static Stretching

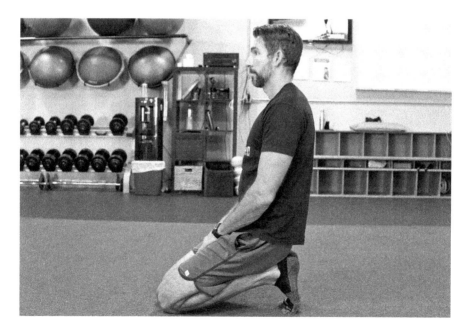

2. Heel Sitting Static Stretching

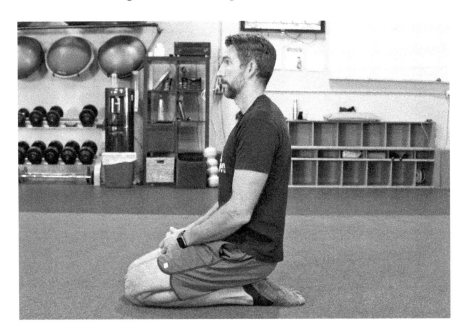

3. Band Assisted Ankle Circles Dynamic Stretch

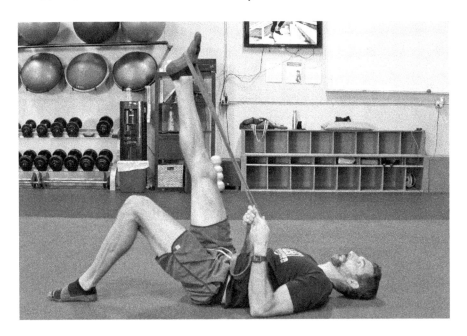

4. KB Anterior Load Half Kneeling Dorsiflexion Stretch

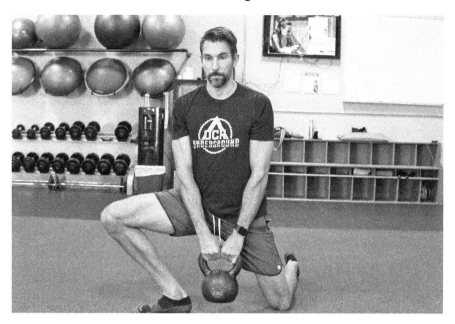

Posterior Hip

5. Band Assisted Hamstring Static Stretch

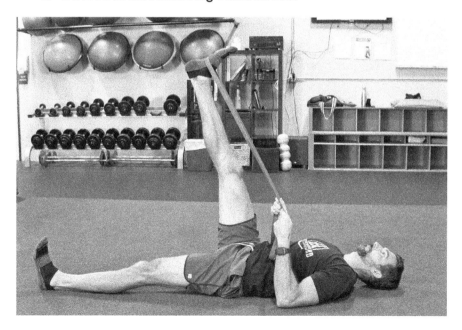

6. Brettzel 2.0 Static Stretch

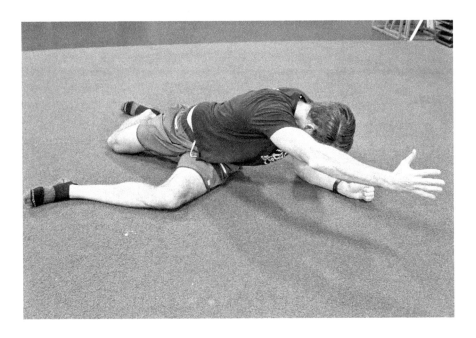

7. Band Assisted Leg Lower Dynamic Stretch

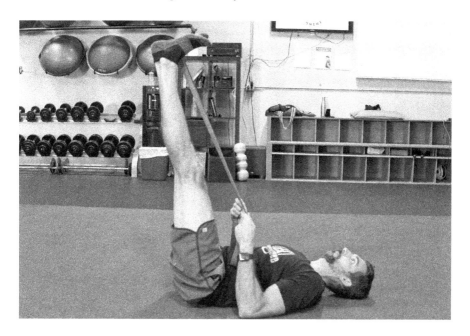

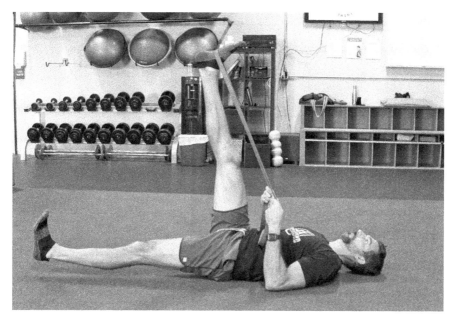

8. 90/90 Rolling Hip Rotation Dynamic Stretch

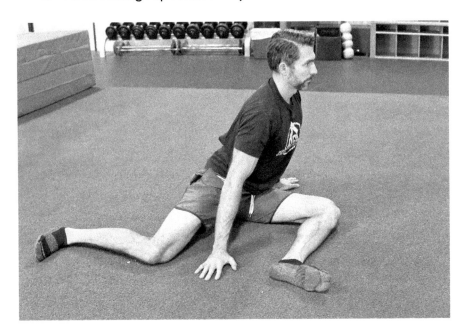

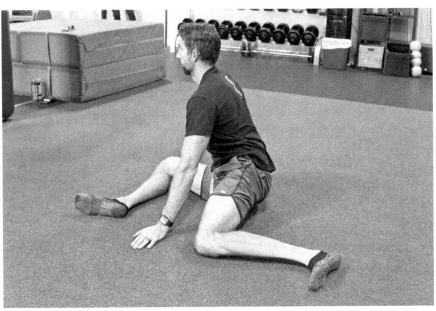

Anterior Hip

9. Rear Foot Elevated Hip Flexor Stretch

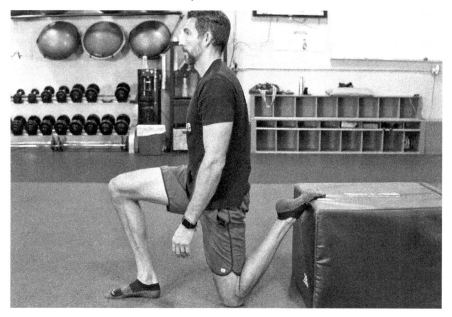

10. Brettzel 1.0 Static Stretch

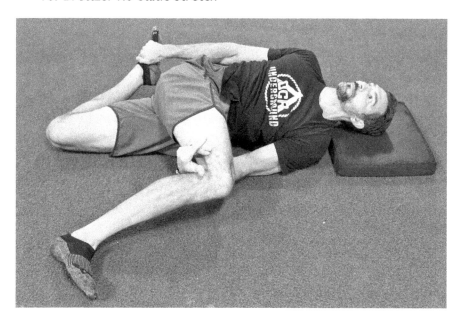

11. Anterior Hip/Posterior Hip Dynamic Stretch

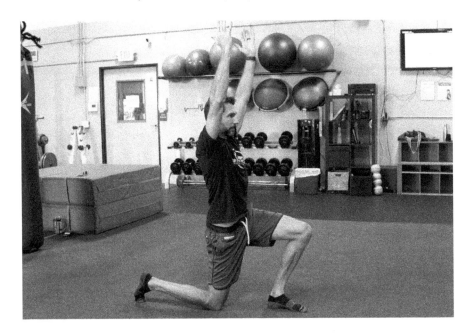

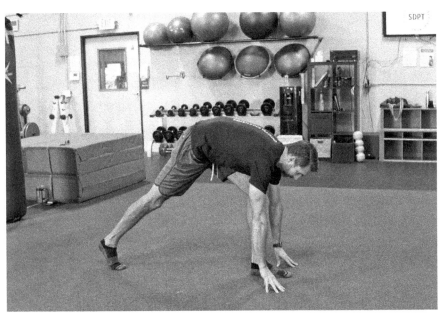

Thoracic Spine

12. Side Lying T-spine Rotation

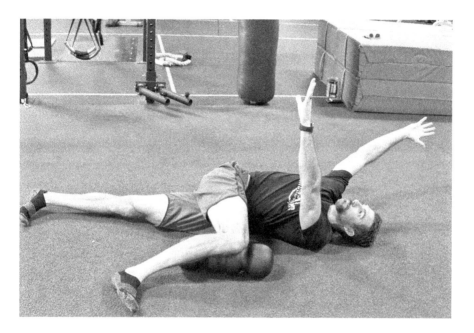

13. Lumbar Lock T-spine Rotation

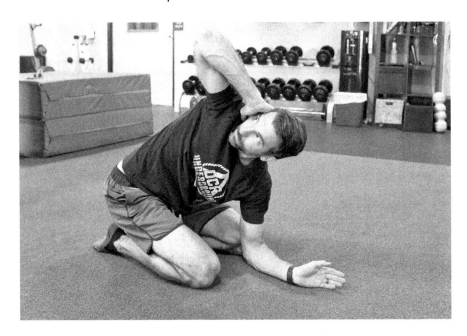

14. Tall Kneeling Posterior Loaded Turns

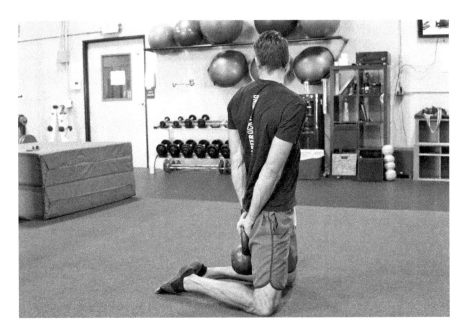

The Shoulder

15. Brettzel 3.0 Static Stretch

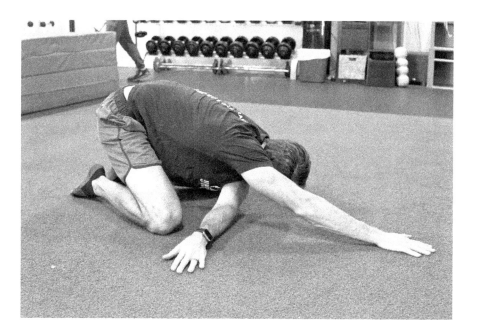

16. Band Assisted 3 Point Shoulder Stretch

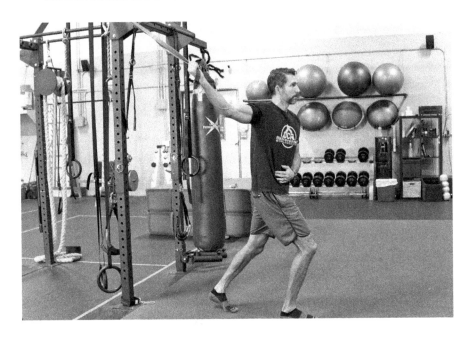

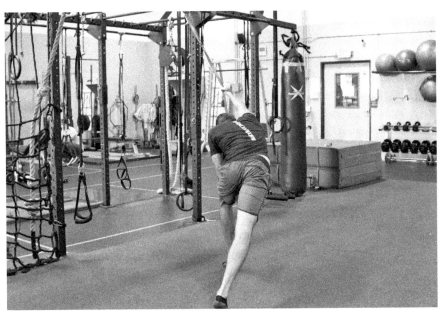

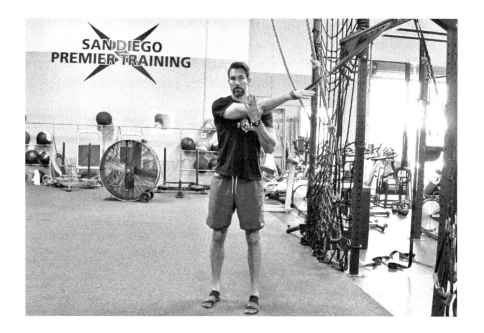

17. Stability Ball Lat Dynamic Stretch

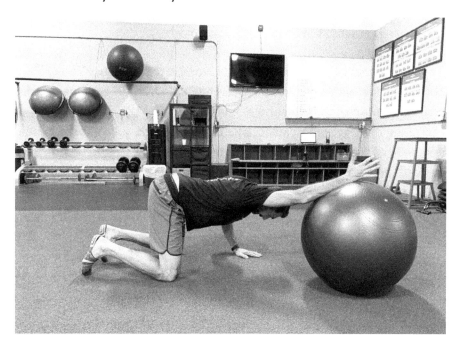

Again, these are a few of my favorite drills that will help improve mobility at each specific joint. It clearly is not every mobility exercise you can do. Find the ones that work best for you. But at a minimum make sure you are at least including one mobility drill for each of the mobility joints.

STABILITY

Stability often has many names associated with it. One example is "activation.".

The goal here is twofold. First, we are doing the best we can to make sure the joint mobility we just improved with rolling is going to stick by strengthening this new range of motion. Second, we are also trying to enhance the control of the stabilizing joints.

So, like the mobility work, we will break exercises down to target each stability joint we are focusing on. Yes, you will have many drills that will cover more than one area, but for our purposes here we will categorize each based on what it may help the most with.

The most important aspect of stability work is to make sure you are not compensating with unwanted movement. We will be training smaller stabilizing muscles to help control joint positions. Make sure you are not recruiting the bigger muscles to take over. Doing so will limit the benefit you will see from these drills. The goal for these exercises is not pure strength. In fact, it does not take much resistance to engage a stabilizer.

Knee Stability Drills

1. Band Resisted Bridges

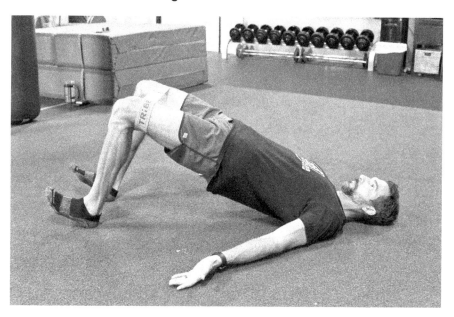

2. Single Leg Bridges

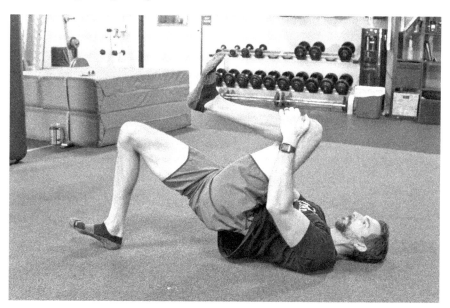

3. Suspension Single Leg Reach

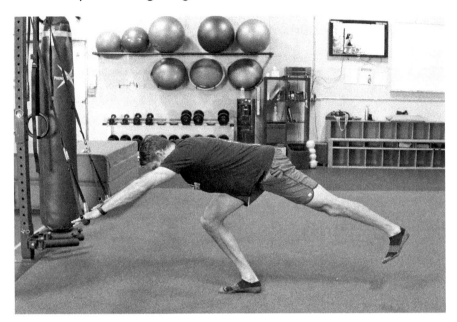

4. Mini Band Walking

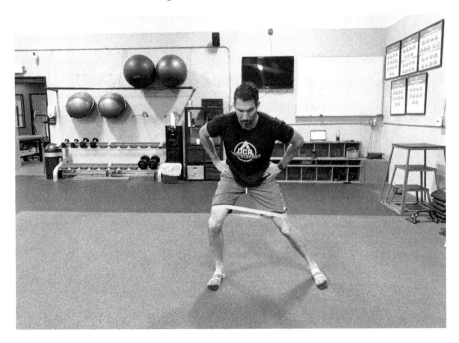

Lumbar Spine Stability Drills

5. Deadbugs

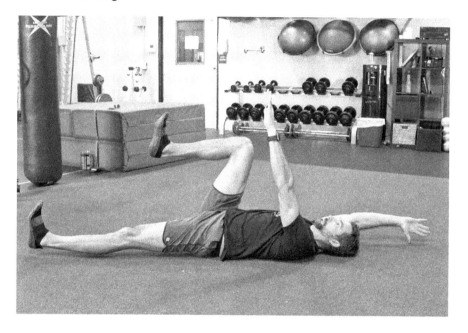

6. Leg Lowering

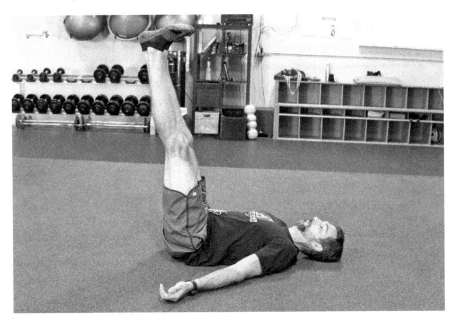

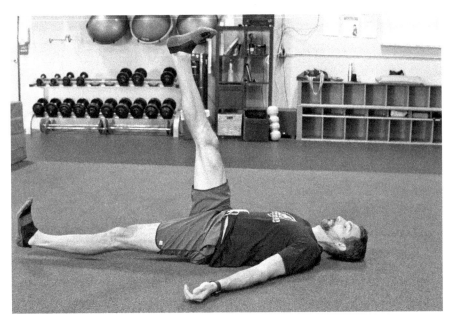

7. Plank

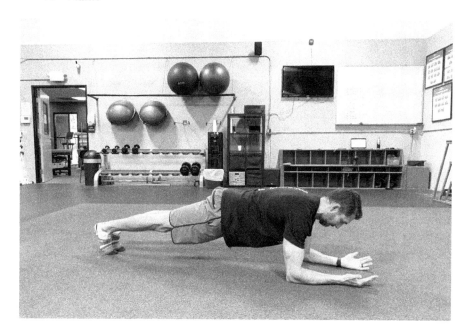

8. Bird Dogs

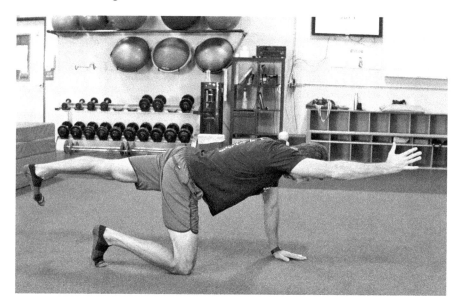

9. Half Kneeling Chop

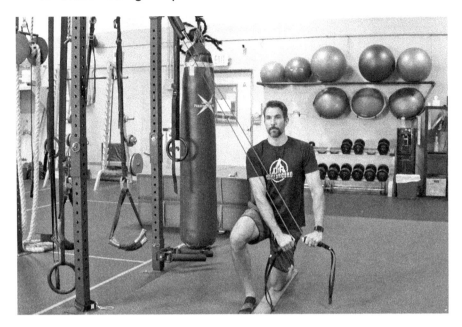

10. Half Kneeling Lift

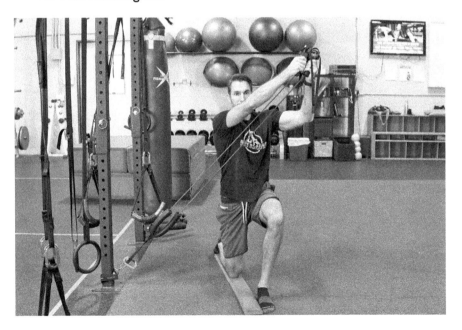

11. Antirotation Press

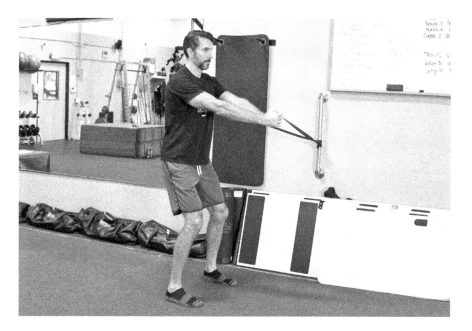

12. Suspension Fallouts

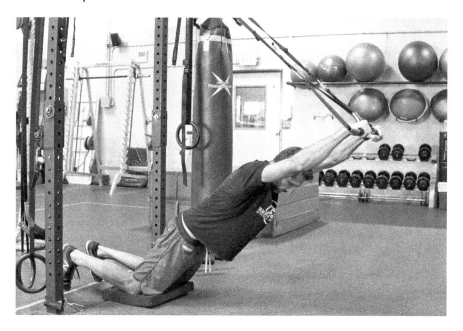

Scapulothoracic Stability

13. Floor Slides

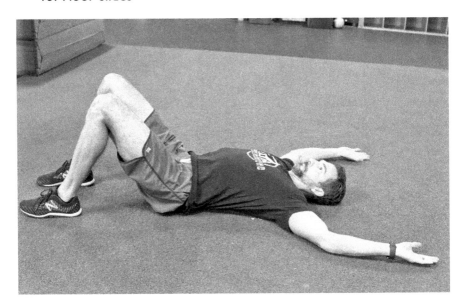

14. ¼ Turkish Get Ups

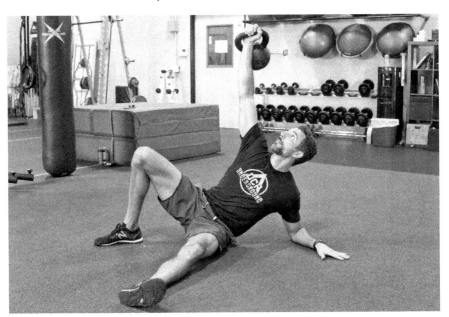

15. Band Pull Apart

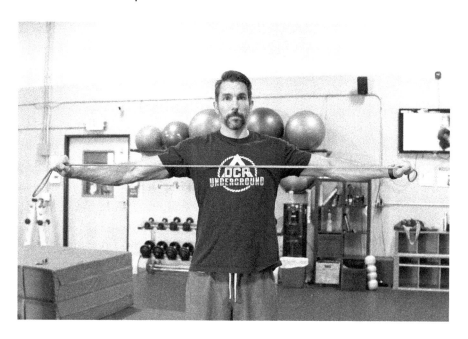

16. Crawling

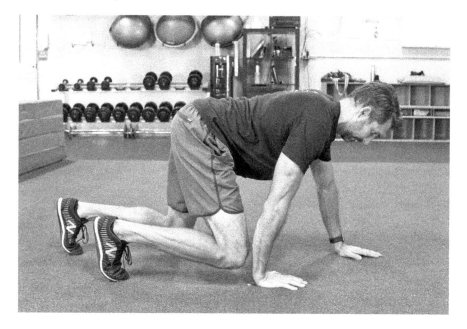

These are just a few variations for stability exercises and, of course, there are hundreds more. This should be a good starting point to see which exercises work best for you. Then you can experiment with other exercises if needed.

CORRECTIVE EXERCISES

This term gets thrown around, probably too much, but we have reached the final piece of our warm-up or movement prep phase. Everything up to this point could be a corrective exercise. But our final piece will be to put all of it together to create better quality movement in the workout.

The corrective exercise section will use the new mobility and stability we just worked on improving to provide better total body movements. You now should have increased ability to perform bigger functional movements so we can do a few drills to make sure you are repatterning efficiently.

There are certain movements that you will perform just about every workout (and throughout every day of your life), so we want to make sure you are getting better at them. Each corrective exercise will be associated with one of these movements. Examples include squatting or lunging.

You may not need to do all of these. You will want to focus on the movement patterns that give you the most difficulty. Think of it as strengthening your weakest link. If they are all weak, then you might want to include more of these exercises:

Hip Hinge Corrective

1. Dowel Assisted Hip Hinge

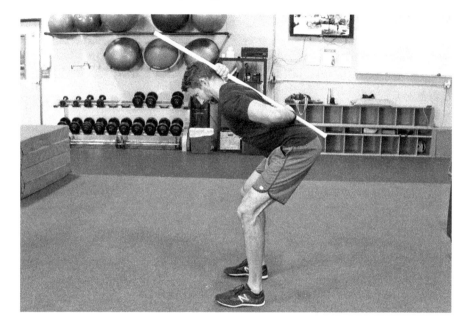

Shoulder Mobility Corrective

2. USB Around the World

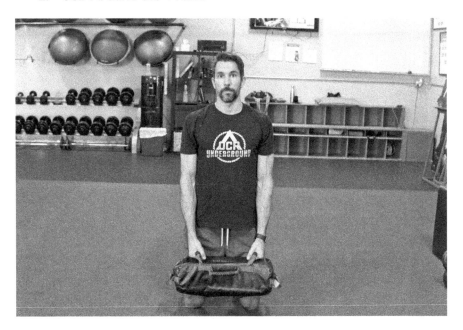

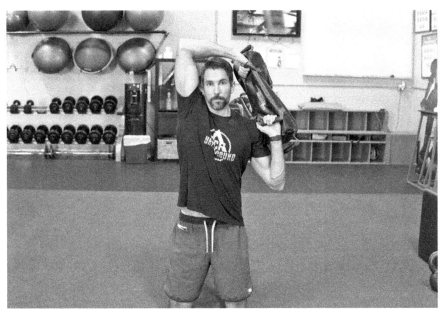

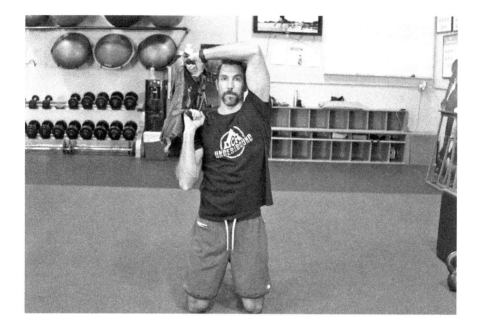

Core Stability Corrective

3. Farmer Carry

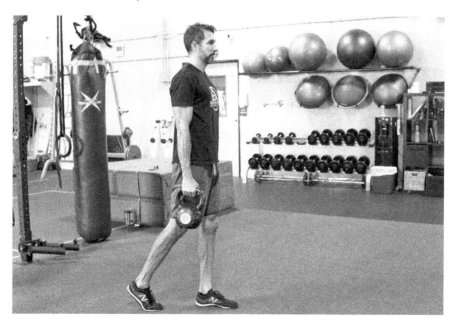

Lunging Corrective

4. Split Squat w/ Band

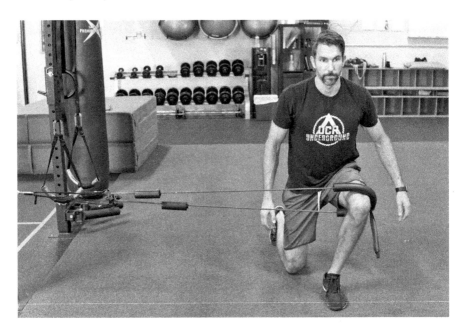

Single Leg Corrective

5. KB Marching

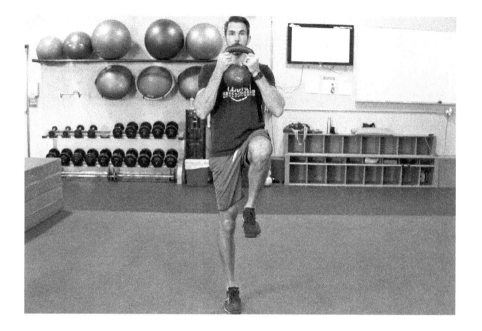

Squatting Corrective

6. Toe Touch Squatting

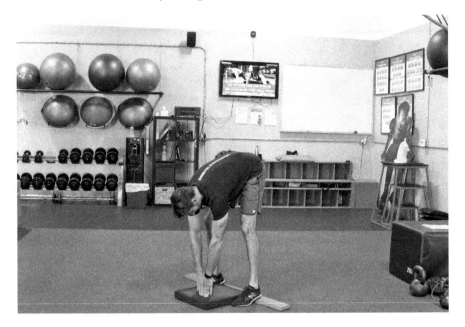

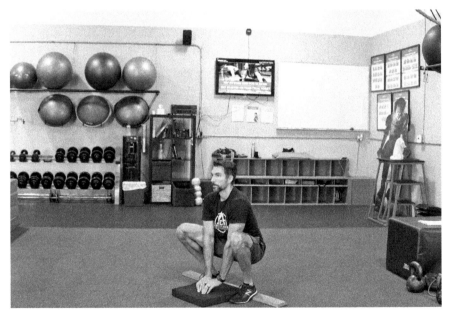

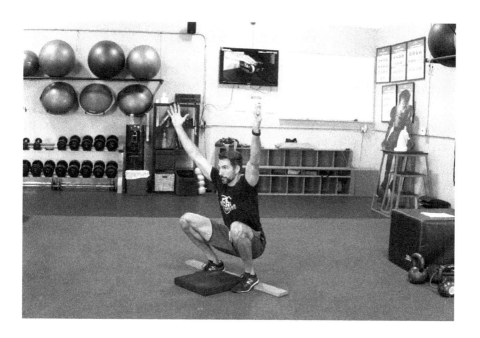

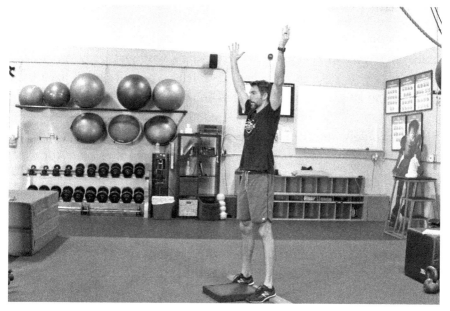

If you have seen the Functional Movement Screen and the correctives associated with it, these will look familiar. As I previously mentioned, if you can find a professional to screen you and give you your specific corrective exercises, you will know exactly where to start.

If not you can use some of these to get an idea of what you could be starting with to help clean up some of your movement patterns.

At this point you should be officially warmed up -- but depending on how conditioned you are --you might feel like you are working out too. That is ok. There is a gray area between the end of the warm up and the start of the workout.

Now we will move on to our power training phase of the workout.

POWER TRAINING

Power training comes in many forms. The idea here is quick movement. Sometimes you will perform power training with just body weight and sometimes you will use both light and heavy tools. They all have their benefits and all should be included in your program.

The classic definition of power is mass times acceleration. In order to create more force or power you can either move more mass (heavier) as quickly as you can or move a smaller mass (lighter) as quickly as you can. Obviously with a lighter mass you can move much quicker. But both are good ways to develop more power.

So why do you need more power? The list goes on and on why we all need power training. But here are a few key points to consider specifically for OCR training.

1. Power will help improve many obstacles you face including running, hill climbing, and wall jumping.

2. Power training works on both acceleration and deceleration of your body and movement. This will better strengthen joints and connective tissue for impact.

3. Power training recruits type IIx muscle fibers. These muscle fibers are much harder to activate with normal training. These are used in order to create the most strength and power with muscle contraction. As other muscle fibers start to fatigue during a race, the more you train these fiber types the more they will be able to help you later in a race.

4. Power training improves your running economy. Numerous studies have shown how lower body power training helps improve running efficiency. This means you use less energy to perform the same running speed. So, runs will become easier for you.

In order to achieve these benefits of power training you must move as quickly as you can. These drills are not conditioning drills, although many can be used for that as well. The goal is to perform high quality, fast reps with adequate recovery. In other words, perform every rep as fast as you possibly can.

To get you started we will demonstrate a few power exercises. Here we can divide them up into 3 categories for training; Upper body medicine ball throws and plyometrics, lower body plyometrics, and power lifts.

UPPER BODY MED BALL THROWS & PLYO DRILLS

Most of our upper body drills will involve medicine ball throws, but there are a few upper body plyometric drills for the more advanced. With medicine ball throws, make sure you are using light med balls. The goal is to move as quickly as you can. When using heavier balls, form begins to deteriorate, and slower movements will occur. Heavier training will be performed with our power lifts, so remember to stick with weights ranging from 2-to-10 pounds.

1. Half Kneeling Rotational Throw

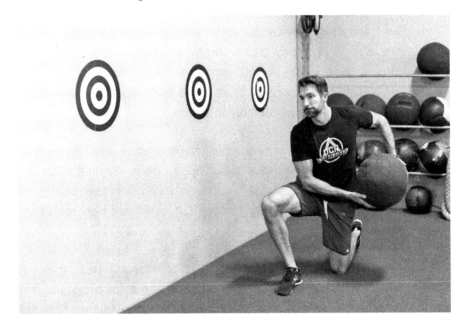

2. Rotational Throw With Step

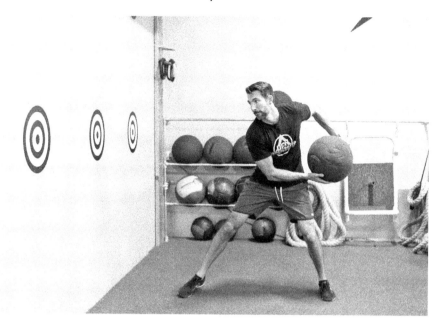

3. Slam

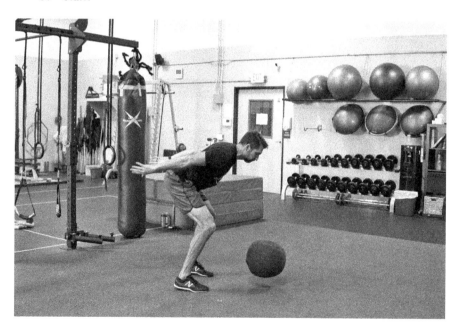

4. Circle Slam

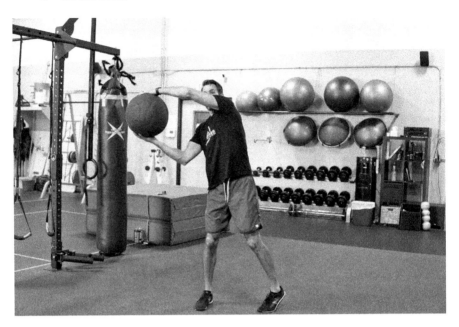

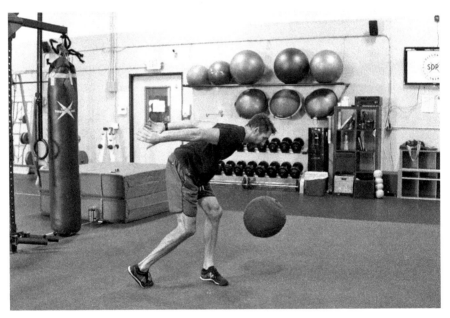

5. Tall Kneeling Chest Throws

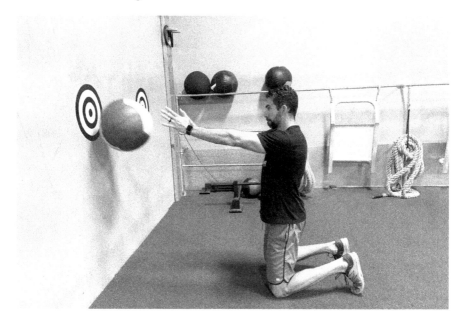

6. Step and Chest Throw

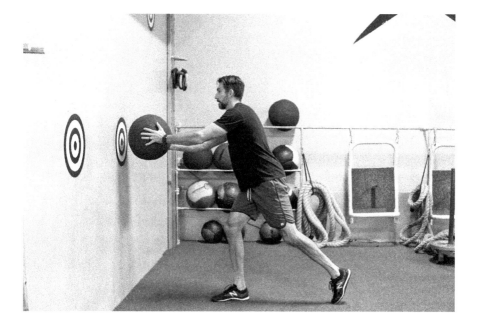

7. Underhand Scoop Toss

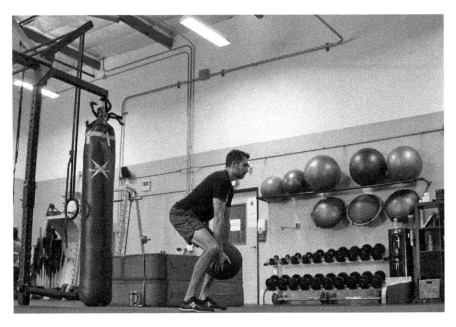

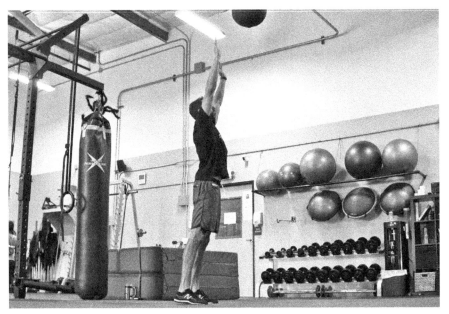

8. Assisted Power Push Up

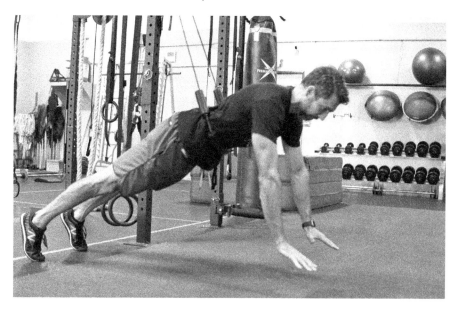

9. MB Power Push Up

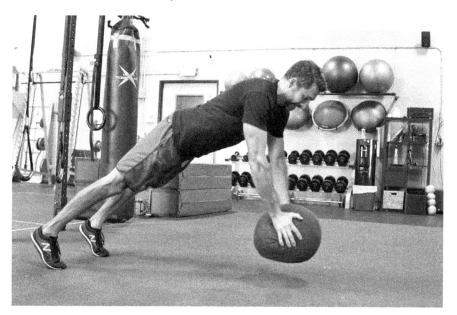

LOWER BODY PLYOMETRICS

Lower body plyometrics are our jumping drills. There is a very simple progression to follow for each set of these drills (created by Mike Boyle).

The first step is to work on landing. You will see a few drills below to help with this. If you can't land properly you shouldn't be jumping.

After you have mastered landing, the next progression is to perform one jump and stick the landing. You will show that you can stabilize the landing before moving on to the next rep. You may feel the urge to skip this step, but I strongly recommend owning the landing for each of these drills.

Once you have shown you can jump and land, we now add a baby jump in between each jump. Essentially you will perform one big jump, then a small jump, then another big jump. The little jump is a way to prepare yourself for the next big jump.

Finally, you will perform consecutive jumps as quickly as you can. Like I mentioned, most just start here, but often lead to injuries because they have not prepared for this type of impact. Plyometrics can be a powerful training tool, but also a way to damage your body if you are not smart about it.

1. Depth Landings

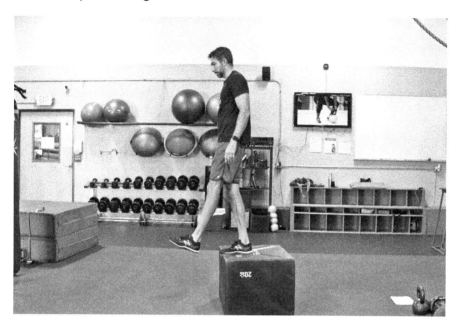

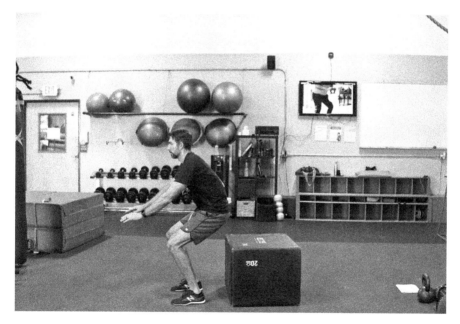

2. Box Jumps

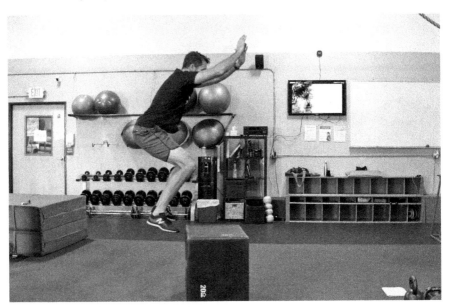

3. Broad Jumps

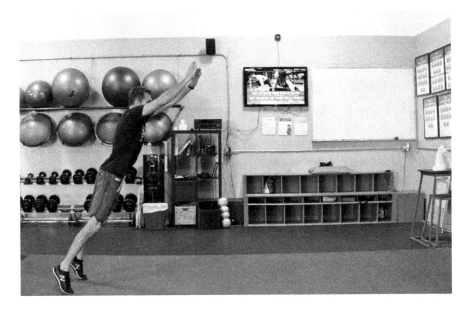

4. Hurdle Jumps

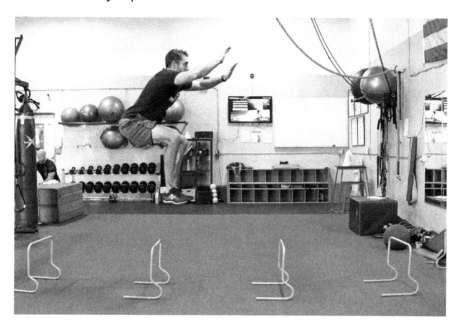

5. Step Jumps

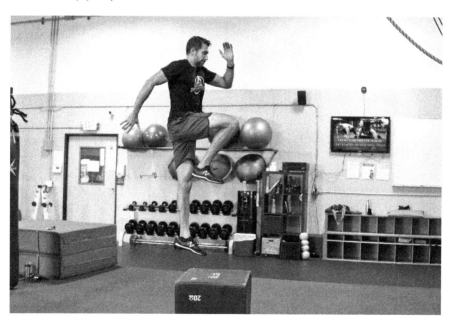

6. Suspension Knee Drives

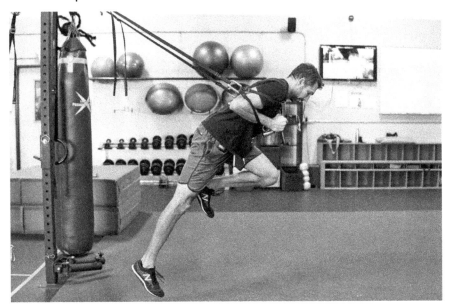

7. 45 Degree Bounds

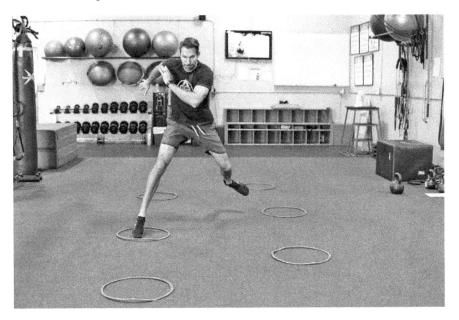

POWERLIFTS

In the previous sections, we discussed performing quick movements using either light implements or body weight. The resistance is fairly light, so your output should be quick movement.

The next series of drills will still involve the intention of moving quickly, but now you will be lifting load. This means the output will be slower. Think of this as a combination of strength training and power. Here you will often see a variety of Olympic lifts, like the power clean and snatch.

Because there is a great deal of skill required to complete these movements, it is a higher-risk activity. For most, I prefer to stick with kettlebells and sandbags rather than loaded barbells. You can still do heavier loads, but with much less risk of injury versus barbells.

Here are some of the most beneficial power lifts you can include.

1. Kettlebell Swings and Single Arm Swings

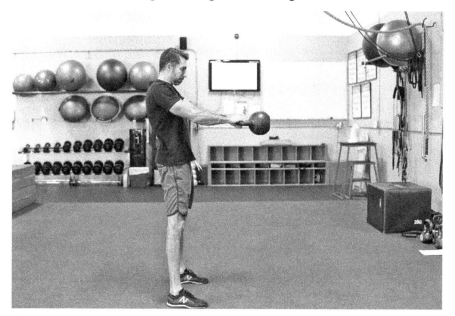

Kettlebell Swing

2. Kettlebell Cleans and Single Arm Cleans

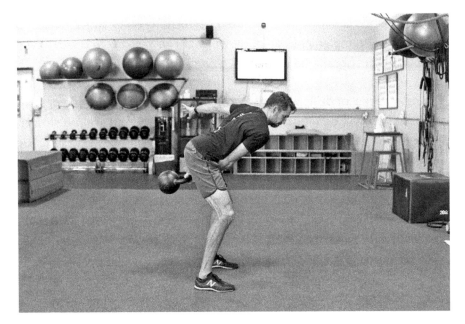

Kettlebell Single Arm Clean

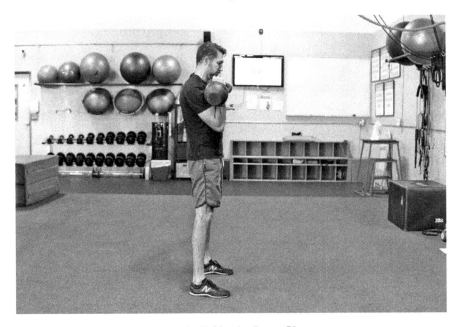

Kettlebell Single Arm Clean

3. Kettlebell Snatches and Single Arm Snatches

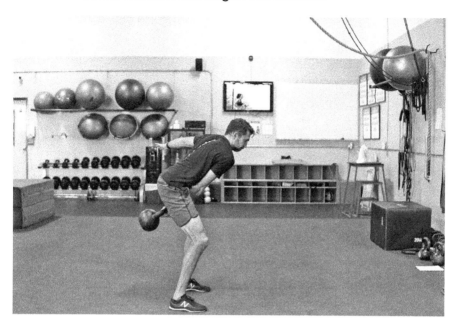

Kettlebell Single Arm Snatch

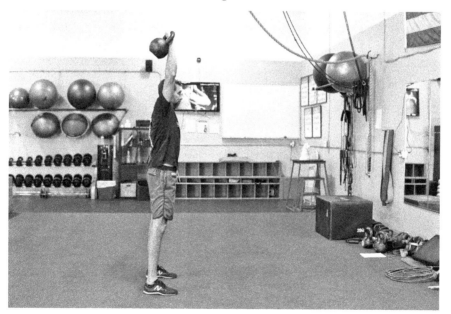

Kettlebell Single Arm Snatch

4. Kettlebell Push Press and Single Arm Push Press

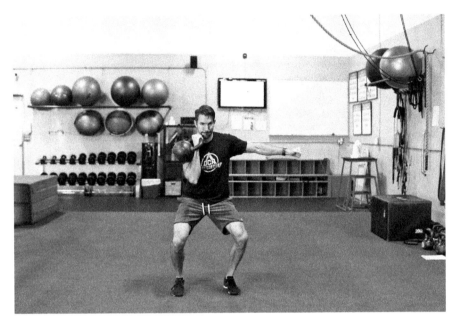

Kettlebell Single Arm Push Press

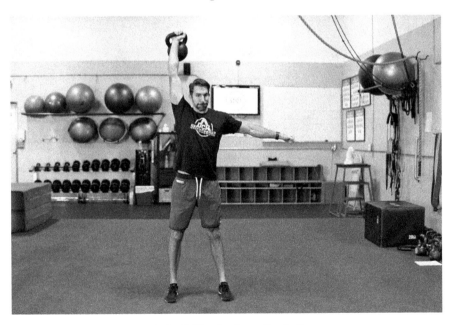

Kettlebell Single Arm Push Press

5. Kettlebell Staggered Stance Single Arm Muscle Clean

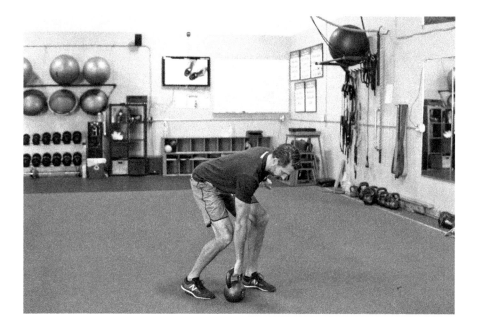

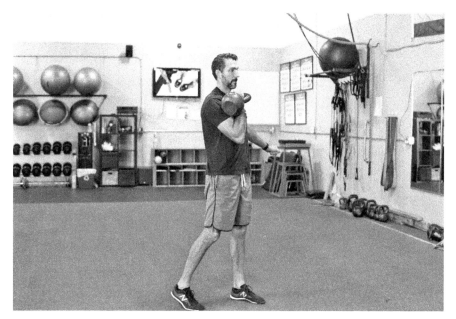

6. Sandbag High Pulls

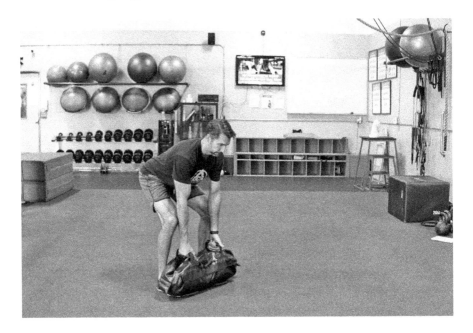

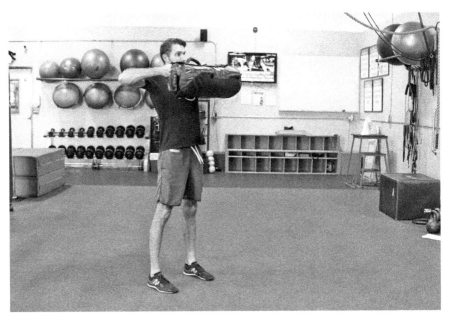

7. Sandbag Clean

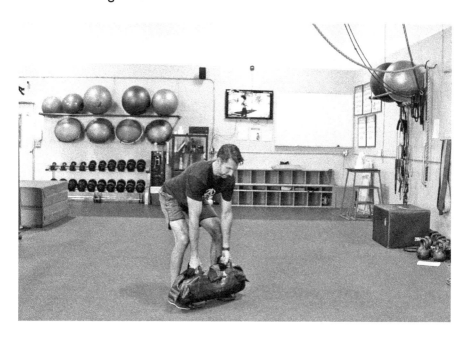

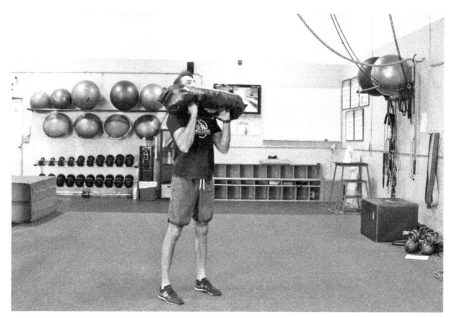

With your power lifts make sure you are keeping the reps between 3-to-6 reps for most exercises, although there are some exceptions. You will want longer recoveries so you can maintain form on each set.

The goal with power moves is quality reps. While there might be a conditioning component to these drills, it is not the goal. Conditioning will be reviewed later. For power training, speed and explosiveness are the most important aspects.

Now let's go get strong.

STRENGTH TRAINING

We have finally arrived at the strength portion of our workout.

We tend to call these workouts strength workouts, but as you will see, there is more than just strength work going on here. This is the key to a comprehensive OCR training plan: You need to be strong, but you need to be mobile and powerful as well.

There are thousands of exercises that you can perform with an effective strength program. We will touch on some of the foundational movements that you need to be doing on a regular basis. My main goal for you in this section is to understand the philosophies we will discuss. This will allow you to create your own programs.

Understanding the guidelines will help you get started, but once you understand how to put together a program you have unlimited options.

To start off, we will review what exercises you should be including. One of the most common mistakes I see when individuals write up a program is they use body part-focused exercises. This is an old school, body-builder style workout. It is great for developing muscle size.

But what is the goal here? Not that bigger muscles won't happen, but our focus is on getting stronger with the goal of increased performance. Following a muscle-focused program will not maximize this effect. If you aren't sure what I am referring to here, a bodybuilding program typically works one or two body parts per day. For example, Monday might be chest day, Tuesday back day, Wednesday leg day, and so on. The problem is the body does not want to move in isolation like this. stop training it this way.

Instead, we will focus on movement patterns. Rather than isolating muscles to maximize growth, you will train the body the way it is supposed to move. In addition to being effective, this is a huge time-saver. You don't need to be doing strength training every day. Two or three days a week of full body training is perfect. Remember, we have other areas of development that are equally important to train on the other days.

Here is the breakdown of movements you will be building your program from.

- Squatting (bilateral and unilateral)

- Lunging or Single Leg Movements

- Hip Hinging (bilateral and unilateral)

- Pushing (bilateral and unilateral/horizontal and vertical)

- Pulling (bilateral and unilateral/horizontal and vertical)

Below you will find just a few examples of each movement pattern. This is to help you get started and give you ideas. Once you understand the pattern there are thousands of variations you can play around with.

The exercises listed are progressive. They start with an easier variation and progress to some of my favorite movements for OCR training.

Squatting

Box Squat

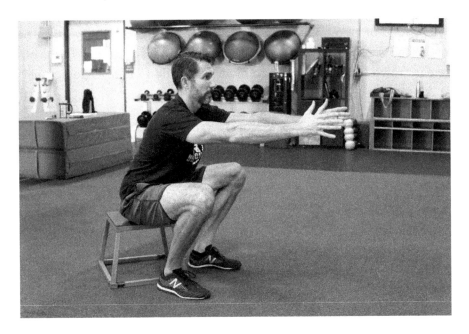

KB Goblet Squat

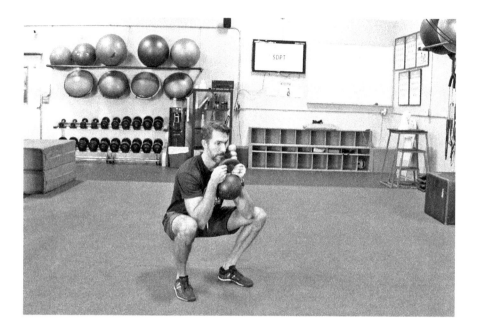

Barbell Front Squat

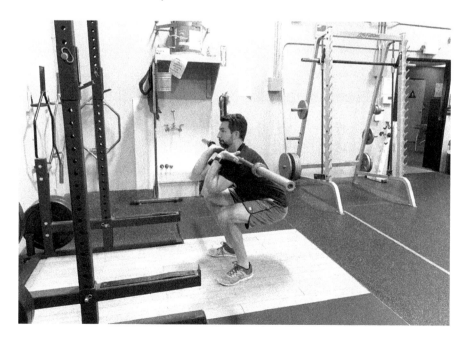

Squatting Single Leg

Assisted Single Leg Squat

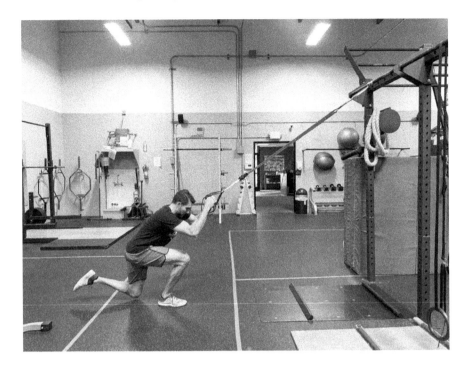

Tennis Ball Single Leg Box Squat

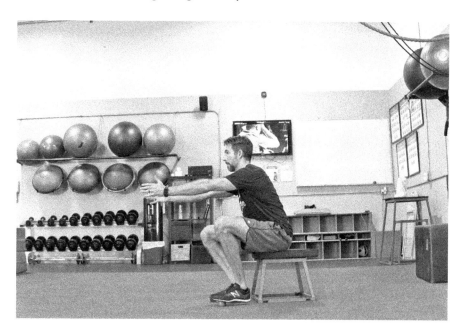

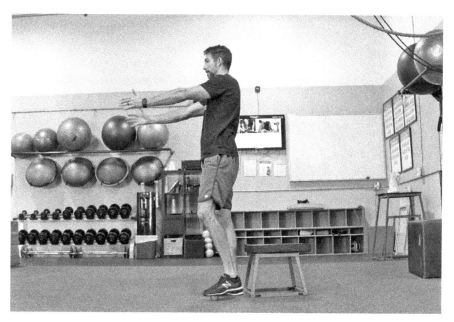

Step to Box Single Leg Squat

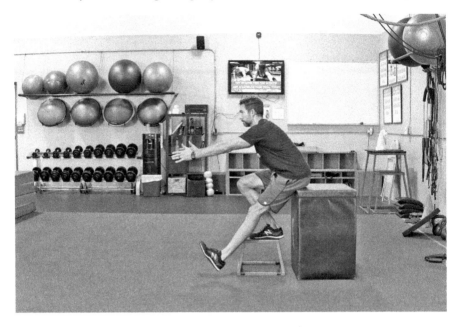

Lunging

Split Squat

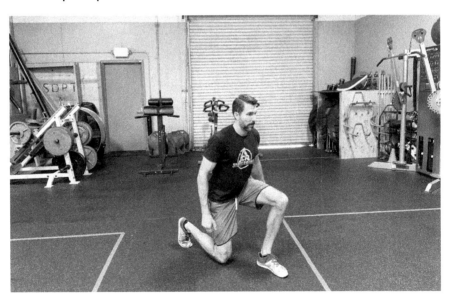

Sandbag Walking Lunge

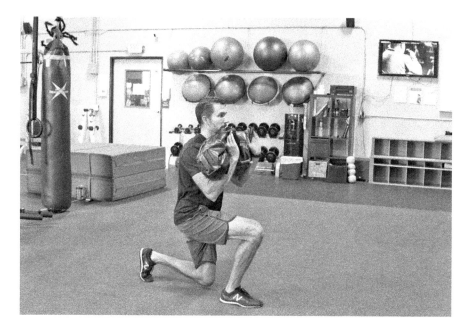

Lunge to Step Up

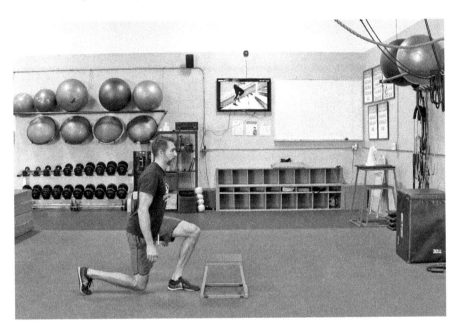

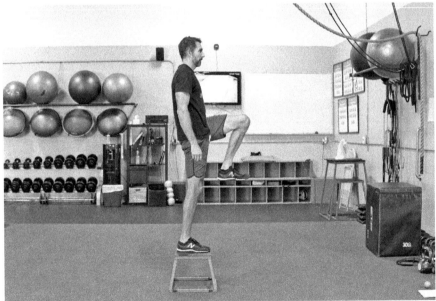

Supine Hip Hinge Drills

Stability Ball Hamstring Curl

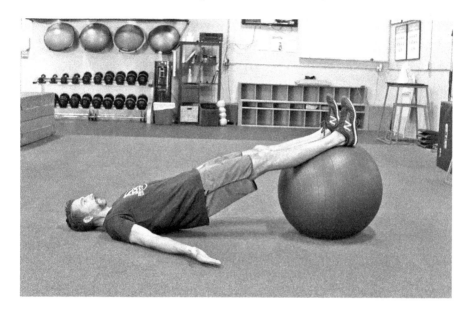

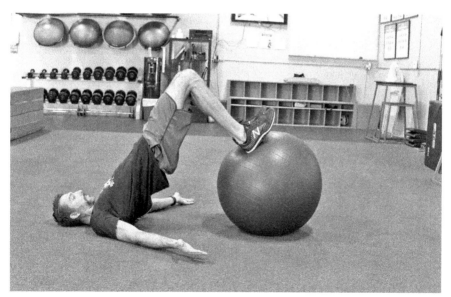

Hip Hinge Drills

Sandbag Good Morning

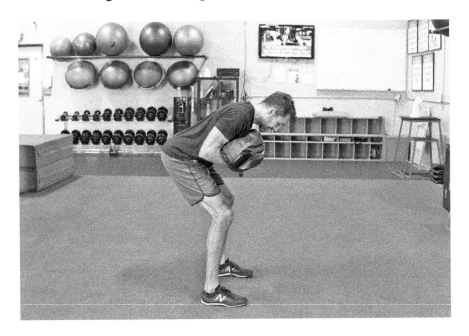

Kettlebell Deadlift

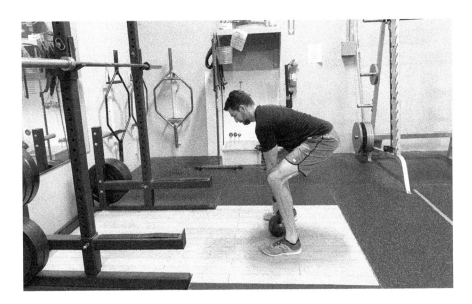

Hexbar Deadlift

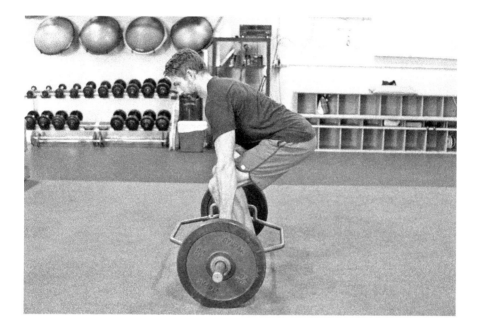

Horizontal Pushing

Push Up Variations

Ring Push Ups

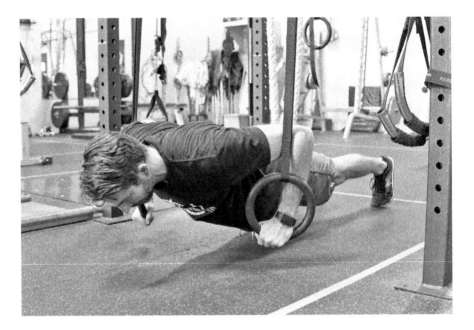

Sliding Push Up

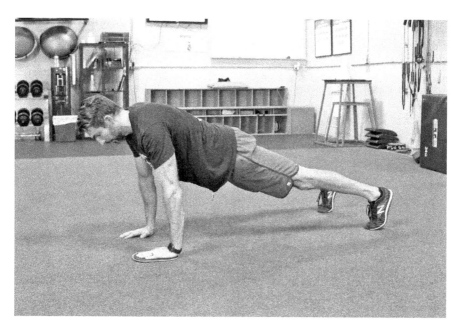

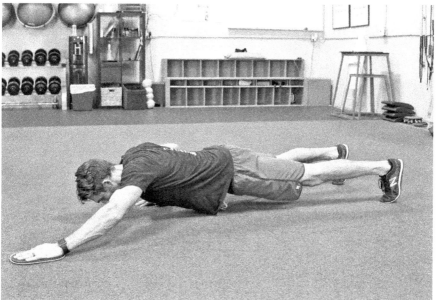

Dumbbell Floor Press

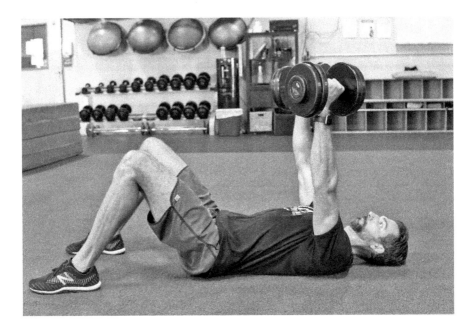

Vertical Pushing

Tall Kneeling Sandbag Pressout (I know this is really horizontal, but for those who can't press overhead this might be a great starting point.)

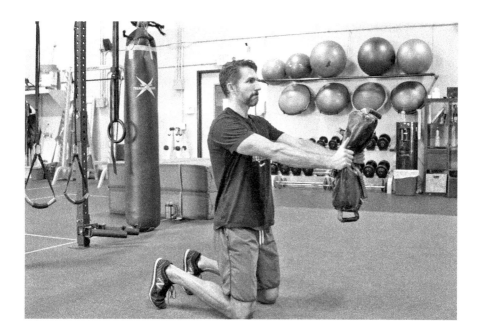

Landmine Half Kneeling Press

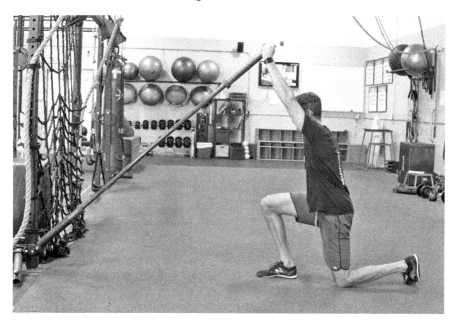

Kettlebell Half Kneeling Bottoms Up Press

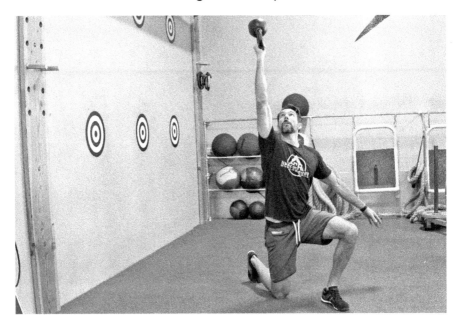

Horizontal Pulling

Inverted Rows

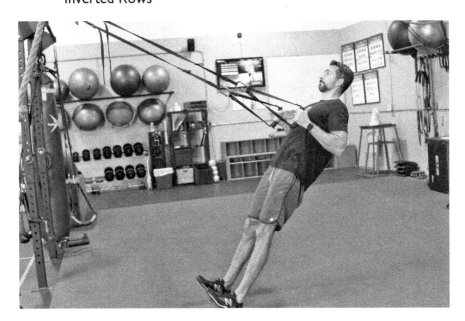

Suspension Trainer Vertical Row

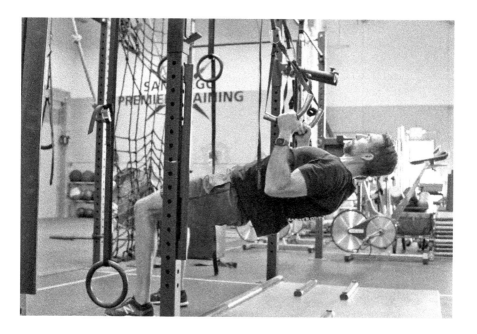

Wide Stance DB Row

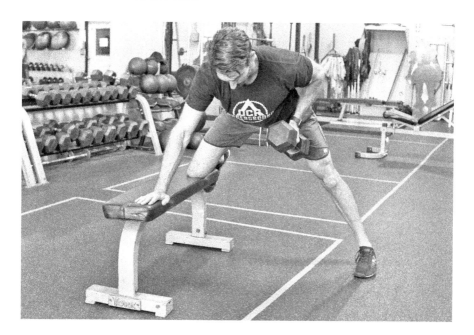

Vertical Pulling

Suspension Pull Ups

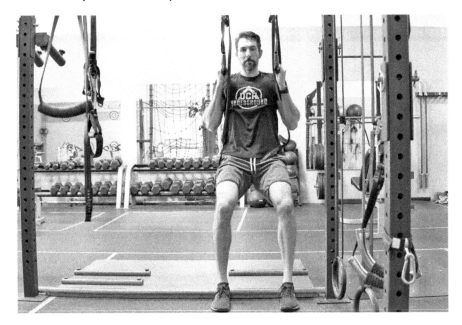

Assisted Pull Ups

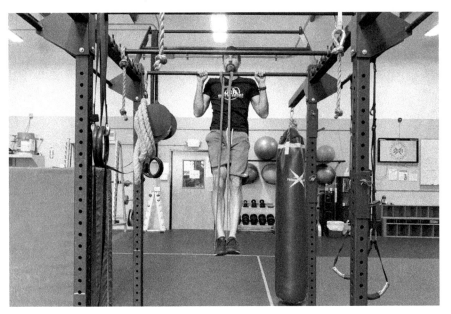

Switch Grip Pull Ups

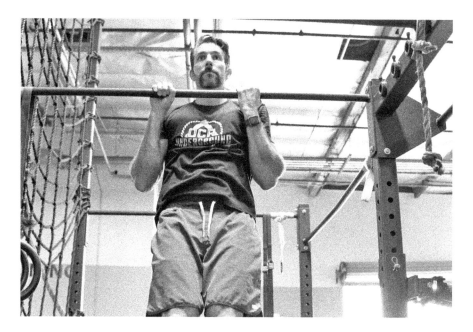

Yes, there are many more options for you, but like any good coach will tell you, your job is to master the fundamentals. Until these are performed effortlessly, with proper technique, you don't have to worry about adding more. Remember, there are videos of each exericse listed above, plus more, at www.ocrunderground.com/book-bonus.

There are a number of ancillary benefits generated by strength training. But the target for these workouts is to get you strong. One mistake that many make is confusing metabolic training or conditioning for strength training. These are separate types of training and have separate goals.

With strength training your priority is to get strong. But how strong do you need to be? In terms of OCR's you only really need so much strength, and at a certain point increased muscle mass will no longer help you. In fact it may hurt performance.

But often athletes need more muscle and to strengthen that muscle. This includes both men and women, but this is possibly more important for women. Indeed, men have an advantage in sports which is why we rarely see men and women competing together. That main advantage is more muscle. So, it only makes sense to do everything you can to get stronger.

Now, how strong? As I just mentioned there is a point where you are no longer seeing a return on your investment. The goal is to get strong enough to perform your best.

This is by no means a perfect science, but experts such as Dan John. Mike Boyle, and Alwyn Cosgrove have come up with strength standards that seem pretty fitting for most individuals. Using some of their numbers and my own experience, here are some numbers to follow as a guideline.

Strength Standards			
Movement	Exercise	Female	Male
Pull	Pull Ups	BW x 3 Reps	BW x 10 Reps
	DB Single Arm Row	.25*BW x 6 Reps Each	.4*BW x 6 Reps Each
Squat	Barbell Back Squat	1*BW x 3 Reps	1.5*BW x 3 Reps
	Barbell Front Squat	.875*BW x 3 Reps	.1*BW x 3 Reps
Hip Hinge	Hexbar Deadlift	1.125*BW x 1 Rep	1.75*BW x 1 Rep
Push	Bench Press	1*BW x 3 Reps	1*BW x 3 Reps
	Push Ups	15 Reps From Toes	30 Reps From Toes
Squat (Single Leg)	DB Rear Foot Elevated Split Squat	30lbs x 3 Reps Each	45lbs x 3 Reps Each
Hip Hinge (Single Leg)	KB Single Leg Deadlift	.4*BW x 5 Reps Each	.5*BW x 5 Reps Each
Total Body	Turkish Get Up	12kg x 1 Rep Each	20kg x 1 Rep Each

To count, each exercise must be executed with great technique and full range of motion. Test your strength for each exercise, if you are ready for this level. If you fall short on any or all of these numbers, you know that strength is going to be a priority.

If you can hit all of these numbers, then you are already at an adequate strength level. This doesn't mean to stop lifting. Instead, your primary focus is now to maintain strength levels or potentially add higher level challenges. There will eventually be a risk-reward relationship that must be examined when trying to get even stronger.

Ok, so now you are getting strong. It is time to finish off your workout.

CONDITIONING

To this point, if you have done everything I have mentioned, you are good to go. You have covered the foundation of any great strength program. But I am also realistic. I know that there are weeks that you will miss some running workouts. You may not get everything in because life just gets in the way.

To compensate, we want to build in a conditioning component to your strength program. This should not be to replace any other conditioning. Think of it as the icing on the cake. Sometimes it's helpful to work on conditioning after you have already completed some lifting. This will help prepare you for the myriad situations you may find yourself in a race.

And let's be honest. Most of my clients love this portion of the workout. I know you too are probably a little crazy and love to torture yourself a bit.

This section will be short with just a few examples of types of conditioning programs you can do. In your workout, you should keep this short and sweet, too. The conditioning workouts are designed to be less than ten minutes long.

These should get you started:

TABATAS

You likely have heard of the Tabata protocol. Tabata workouts are very intense, with a cycle of 20 seconds hard effort followed by 10 seconds recovery, for a total of eight rounds. I must admit Tabata training has been blown a bit out of proportion in terms of the results it will yield, but still I think it is an effective tool for short conditioning work.

Try using four different exercises with the 20-second on/10-second off intervals for two rounds. You will be done in four minutes. You can add more sets as you build up your fitness.

Sample Tabata Set

KB Swings

Battling Rope Waves

Burpees

Med Ball Slams

SLED PUSHING

Along with other valuable benefits, pushing a heavy sled can definitely build conditioning. This is pretty straight forward. Load up a sled with a challenging weight and push. You can use a variety of positions and handles based on the type of sled you have, but they all work well.

The main thing to focus on is, even though we are training conditioning, don't throw form out the window. You should be concentrating on your posture the entire time you are pushing. Some good areas to focus on are keeping your chest tall, not stepping too far in front of you, and driving your feet into the floor. This will help you produce better force and improve your running form at the same time.

Shoot for four-to-six rounds of pushes, each push around 30-to-40 yards each. If you are wearing a heart rate monitor you can rest until your HR returns to around 70% before you perform your next push.

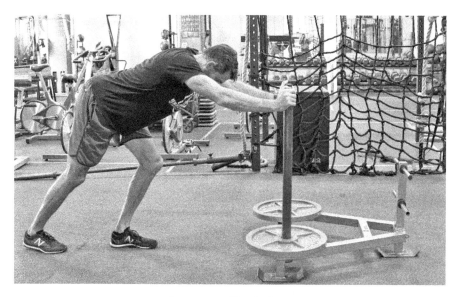

Improper Technique

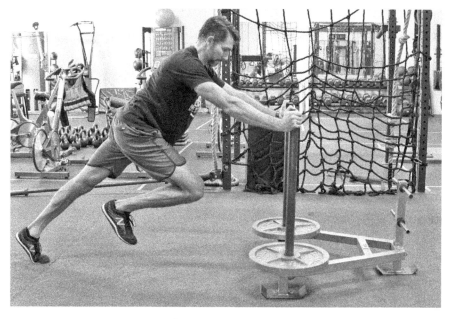

Proper Technique

ASSAULT BIKE

We saved the best for last. Most people have a love-hate relationship with Air Bikes. There are many different brands out there, but I am most familiar with the Assault Bike, so I'll use this brand for my example.

The two most potent ways you can use the bikes are with intervals and tempo rides. Intervals can vary using time or distance. To get started try using 10 seconds bursts and build up to 30-to-60 second sprints. Then using your heart rate as a guide, wait until it lowers to 70-75% and repeat for 4-6 rounds.

You can also perform tempo rides on the Assault Bike. This is essentially riding a certain distance as fast as you can.

It is good to follow a progression with tempo rides. Start with one mile and slowly progress up to five miles. These should be performed at the highest intensity you can maintain, so keep track of your time. This will give you a goal for the next time you perform this workout.

PERIODIZATION

Now that you have an understanding of the workouts you will perform to build strength, we have to talk about periodization. This is a fancy word for planning your year.

You can't train the same way all the time. Even though this is what most people will do, it is only going to work for a short period and then you will see a massive stall in your progress.

This can be a complicated topic, but we will keep it simple discussing the essential points you will need. The easiest way I have found to periodize a program is with an off-season and in-season training plan.

This is tough because most athletes are racing all year and won't have a traditional off season like most sports will. But we still can't try and peak for every single race you are doing. Certain times of the year are most likely going to be more important than others. Or maybe there's a particular race that you are hoping to do really well at.

This doesn't mean you aren't going to train for every race and try to do the best you can at every race. It is more about prioritizing certain races.

This accomplishes a few things. It helps you peak at the right time for the right race or races, plus it keeps you from getting in your own way. One of the biggest problems athletes run into is overtraining and/or beating up their body too much.

OCR can be very hard on the body. Races alone can beat you up, so why have a training program that is going to do the same? I have seen so many athletes run themselves into the ground with their training plan and never get to do the races they were training for.

Don't let this happen to you. Be smart with your training and have a system to follow.

I will usually pick a few months of the year that are right after my most important races. This will start my off-season. The main goals during this period are to work on any areas of weakness, recover from any injuries from the season, back off mileage and crosstrain, dial in technique and form during training, and get strong.

You want to finish your off season feeling great. You should be recovered from the prior season, yet building massive strength to help build a solid foundation to stack the rest of your training on top of.

To set up strength workouts you can use a linear periodization program. This means you start with lower intensity and build up progressively each phase. For example, phase I you may be using loads you can handle for 15 reps; phase 2 loads for 12 reps; phase 3 loads for 8 reps; and phase 4 loads for 6 reps. This is more a traditional training model.

Once you complete your off-season you then progress into your in-season plan. Now you will focus on more specific obstacle training with your tactical work. This will be covered in detail in the next section. You will also now increase your mileage and start more race-specific running workouts. For your strength programs you will follow what is called an undulating periodization model. This means you will be varying rep ranges week to week or even workout to workout.

You will not maximize any one area of emphasis, but instead do everything you can to maintain as much power, strength, and endurance as you can at the same time. You will see examples in our sample program to get you started. One way to set up this type of training is to divide your weekly strength workouts into a strength day, muscle-building day, and endurance day. This may look like 4-6 reps on day one, 8-12 on day two, and 12-15 reps on day three. This way each week you are hitting different strength goals.

Now that we have covered your strength routines, let's look at the obstacle specific training.

CHAPTER 7

TACTICAL TRAINING

Tactical Training is any specific work used to help improve your racing skills. Here you will perform workouts that are designed to simulate race conditions or train for specific obstacles.

This can be a huge challenge since it's likely you don't have access to actual obstacles to train on. Some have solved this problem by building courses in their backyards. Also, it's now possible to find gyms that have obstacles to practice on. Great solutions, but for many these may not be options.

Instead we are going to focus on things you can easily do to help with specific race skills. At the end of the book I will share a few of my favorite tactical workouts you can do with minimal equipment. But first we will review some of the essentials in programming and movements.

Programming is pretty simple. These workouts are hard. They should be pushing you to the limit -- since that is what most races are going to do.

I will be honest. Most of my clients _love_ these workouts. These workouts will push you. With that in mind, my suggestion is to be cautious; limit these types of workouts to once or twice per week. Because of the demands they place on athletes, we often see injuries pop up when this becomes the focus of your training.

There is a specific reason we are talking about tactical last. While it is important, your strength and running will make up the bulk of your training plan. If you don't have strength and running laid down as a foundation, you won't see much improvement in your ability to handle obstacles.

Let's now cover the main movements that you will focus on for your tactical training. These include running, crawling, climbing, jumping, and carrying. These are primal movement patterns that are essential for obstacle course racing.

RUNNING

We have already covered much of your run training earlier in the cardiorespiratory training chapter. Your focus with running is race-specific training. What I mean by that is you will negotiate obstacles after running at race-pace speeds, so you are out of breath and fatigued.

You will also run <u>after</u> completing obstacles. So it's equally important to train yourself to recover your race pace after completing an obstacle.

Your form and breathing will be critical. The goal is to hit higher intensity runs, both flat and on the hills, but not lose control of your breathing and not lose control of your running form. If this means initially you have to slow down your pacing, that is ok. You will adapt quickly and be able to pick it up.

Primarily stick with higher intensity zone runs. Depending on what race length you are training for, your distances will vary, but you will include anywhere from short 30-second hill sprints to longer one-mile hard runs. These runs will be used to break up the obstacle-specific workout you will be doing.

Complete books and programs have been created on improving your running form. This will go beyond the scope of this book, but you can check out programs like Pose or Chi running. To get you started on improving your running technique, I recommend simply doing your running warm up barefoot on a safe surface. Barefoot running is a great self-limiting exercise. This means when you do it wrong you will know. It forces you to take smaller, quicker strides and midfoot strike, which are some of the biggest concerns in running.

CRAWLING

In most races you will have to get down and do some crawling, so it makes sense that we see crawling patterns here. But these types of exercises are not just to get you ready for a barbed wire crawl (although it will help). These exercises will also help improve your core strength as you become more efficient at the crawling pattern. Crawling is how we originally learned how to walk, then eventually run. You would be amazed at how many runners can't crawl properly. This means these runners cannot coordinate opposite arm and leg movement while controlling force with their core.

Coordination and form will be the focus of your crawling for your tactical workouts. You learn to use the core properly and coordinate upper and lower body movement simultaneously. Yes, you will go slower and yes, it will make these drills harder. But it will pay off in the long run.

The main goal I want you to focus on is moving your arm and leg together. That means the right arm and the left foot leave the ground, and make contact again, at the same time. It should be one, fluid movement.

Your contact points should also be emphasized. Most athletes will only focus on the arm and leg moving. While I want you to make sure they move together, you must also focus on creating force with your contact points. You will do this by pushing into the ground as hard as you can. This will be the source of your stability and allow you to learn how to use your core properly.

To tell if you are doing it right, try putting a yoga block or other light object on your back. You should be able to do any type of crawl without it falling off. If you feel your hips moving side to side, you have lost proper stability.

Here are several crawling movements to make progress on:.

Bear Plank

Crawl in Place

Bear Crawl

Reverse Bear Crawl

Lateral Crawl

CLIMBING

Luckily, even if you don't have obstacles to climb over or on in your training, crawling is the foundation for climbing.

Imagine someone crawling and they flip their body position 90 degrees vertically, they would be climbing.

So, the rudiments of the movements are the same; it's simply a matter of making some changes in the muscles that will need to be strengthened. For instance, we are going to use hanging exercises to bolster your climbing. It is not precisely the same, but if you have limited equipment, these will be your go-to exercises for the climbing pattern.

With each of these drills, it will be important to keep shoulder and hip position in mind. The problem is these drills are very difficult for most, and many will develop compensations to try and hang on for longer. For your shoulder, you must keep it packed or close to the joint -- like the opposite of a shrug. You will want to push your shoulders down and away from your ears as you hang. For your hips, you want to do the best you can to maintain the hollow hold position.

If you imagine your pelvis as a bucket of water, you do not want any water to spill out. Most will allow the hips to rotate forward when they hang. This will put increased pressure on your lower back.

Here are a few progressions to help with your hanging.

Hollow holds

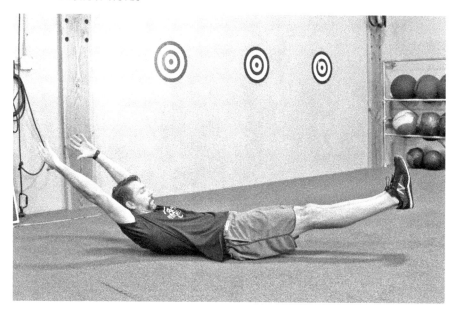

Horizontal Hangs

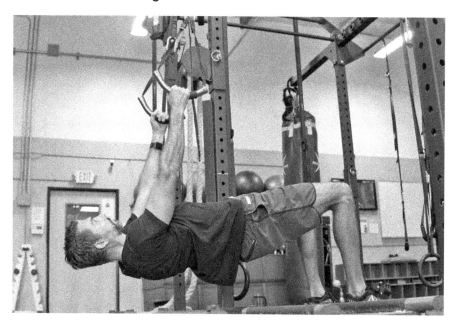

Dead Hang

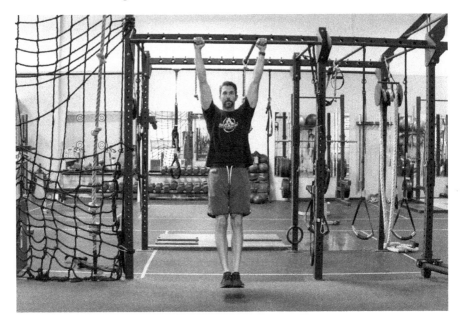

Dead Hang Marching

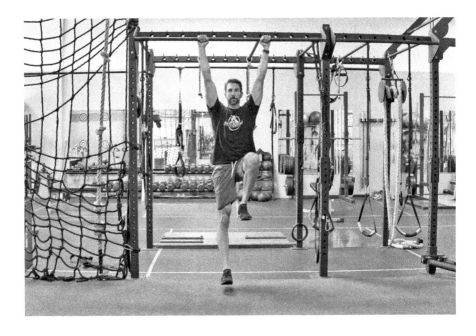

Alternating Hangs

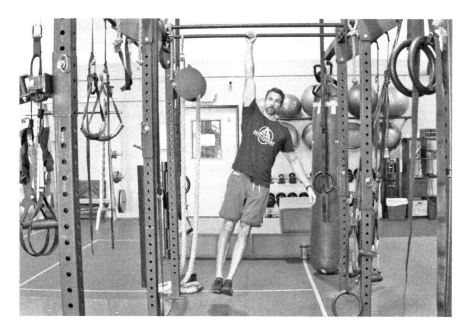

JUMPING

We've talked about jumping but it will be valuable to include here as we work on obstacles like wall climbs. The more power you can generate, the easier time you will have getting over these obstacles. The main point is to include both single leg and double leg jumping drills as you will likely need both for different obstacles you face.

CARRYING

Carrying can seem straight forward. You grab a heavy weight and go for a walk. As simple as these exercises can be, if you perform them correctly you will receive an incredible array of benefits. The mistake most often made is not understanding the essential techniques for carrying.

The first step is understanding this is a postural loading exercise. The goal is to be able to maintain a good posture while carrying a load. If you round your shoulders and back -- while shooting your head forward --you are training the wrong muscles to do the work.

The skeletal structure should be taking most of the weight, while your stabilizing muscles do the rest. It is a good idea to start with marching drills to make sure you can maintain a good posture. This means your ears are over your shoulders, which are over your hips. Maintain this alignment while walking. If you cannot, lower the weight and rest. Always reinforce good position.

Since this is a postural and stabilizing exercise, you should be using minimal effort. Carrying for long times will lead to fatigue all over, but initially it should not take much effort. If you were wearing a heart-rate monitor we would see very low heart rates during carries, until maybe the very end. If you immediately jump to a high heart rate, you are using an upper threshold strategy, indicating that you are using the wrong muscles to carry the weight.

To help you with this, here are some of the best cues I can use to reinforce good technique.

- First, hold the weight -- do not lift it. If you start to feel your upper trapezius and neck fatiguing you are probably using the wrong muscles to carry the weight. When holding the weights at your side imagine trying to press the weights to the floor. This should cause an anti-shrug movement, helping maintain proper shoulder alignment.
- Next, it is important to use your latissimus dorsi. This muscle is incredibly important for supporting your carries and saving your grip. To make sure you are using your lats, imagine you have a $100 bill in each armpit. As you walk do not let the bills fall out. This image usually helps get the correct muscles working.

Here are some of my favorite carrying progressions. Below there are a few sample pictures, but make sure you visit www.ocrunderground.com/book-bonus for complete exercise demonstration of each and tutorials.

KB Goblet Marching

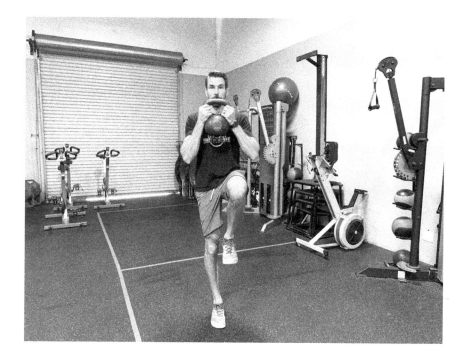

KB Goblet Carry

Sandbag Carry

KB Single Arm Carry

KB Double Arm Carry

KB Racked Carry

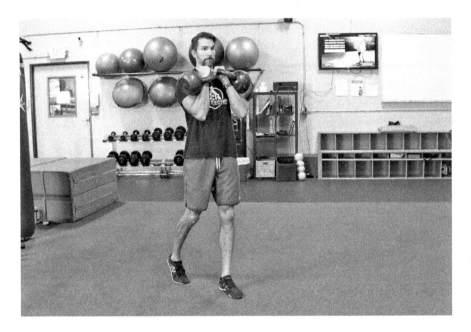

Bucket Carry

KB Overhead Carry

6 Point Carry Drill

ADDITIONAL TACTICAL WORK

Everything mentioned so far should comprise the bulk of your tactical training, but there are many other items we can also add in. You will find videos of each tactical training exercise at www.ocrunderground.com/book-bonus.

SPECIFIC OBSTACLE WORK

Yes, we can get on obstacles when available. There is a technique to each of them. But if you are strong you should be able to get through most obstacles. This is why I make strength the emphasis. If you do not have enough strength, technique won't save you.

If you want help on specific obstacles and techniques to get through them, you can check out my 90 Day Fuel and Fire Program at https://ocrunderground.com/programs/.

BURPEES

I have mixed feelings on burpees. Like in Spartan Races, you'll find them implanted into many OCR events, so burpess are important to practice. It can also be used as a conditioning drill, but it is often abused. I cringe a bit when I see burpee challenges up online. Repeatedly throwing yourself down on the floor can lead to many issues, so use burpees sparingly. And when you perform burpees make sure you understand and emphasize good technique . Don't be ashamed to do them on an incline to work on your form.

HILL SPRINTS

Running was already mentioned, but hill sprints are a great way to work on conditioning and your running at the same time. There is nothing quite like sprinting up hills as hard as you can. You will hate it, but you will love the results.

Don't have access to hills? While not the same, there are a few things you can do here to substitute. If you have a spin bike, try bumping up the resistance until you can only manage an RPM of 25-30. Maintain this pace for 2-5 minutes.

ASSAULT BIKE

I had to bring this one up again. If you have seen an Assault Bike, they are the bikes with the big fan on the front. I love these for a few reasons. One, it is low impact. Not many activities can get your heart rate up like this with minimal impact on your joints. Those with injuries and unable to run will get a lot of benefit from the bike. This is true of many bikes on the market, but with this type we have the added benefit of incorporating the upper body making it a total body exercise. Plus, the wind resistance is a great addition.

It also gives you a break from running. So many injuries arise from over-training with running. Why not take a few breaks and cross-train on the bike?

LUNGES

I know we previously covered lunging, but sometimes you can't get out on the hills to train for a race. If hills are inaccessible, lunges are an excellent substitute. They will strengthen the legs and help you prepare for races with hill climbs. Add bucket and sandbag carries to your lunge drills for even more of a good time.

That wraps up everything you need for your physical training for your race. To finish up the book we will cover your nutritional support and mental training.

CHAPTER 8

NUTRITION

Entire books have been devoted to nutrition and its role in athletic performance. We will only have one short chapter to squeeze this subject in. Hopefully this works toward your benefit and eliminates the complexity and confusion that often surrounds discussion on what to eat.

You probably already know there are different macronutrients, like fats, carbohydrates and proteins, that you need to get into your diet. These topics will be covered but hopefully in a more practical sense. We will keep it to the point and focus on what you need to do to optimally fuel your body to be efficient.

Efficiency is the key we need to talk about. This is something that takes time. Do not expect any magic to happen immediately. We will manipulate your diet to help your body run the way it was designed, but these adaptations take time. And sometimes you will struggle in the beginning. Hang in there. It will all be worth it.

To start, let us make sure we focus on the right goal. For example, you may have some weight you are trying to lose. While improved body composition may be a side product of this nutrition plan, it is not the priority. Instead, we are focusing on performance.

If you are trying to lose body fat, you must be in a caloric deficit. Any time you are not getting enough calories to support your activity, there will be a drop in performance. So if weight management is your priority, you will still benefit from this chapter, but just remember this is not a program targeted at weight loss. Weight loss may still occur as a side product of this plan depending on where you are starting from. But if you are not at your ideal or close to your ideal weight, that should be a priority.

The next question that comes up involves the type of diet you should follow, plant-based, vegan, keto, etc. I am not going to get into these specific details. To be honest, if you talk to a plant-based enthusiast, they will only show you the data that makes that style of eating sound awesome. And vice versa, if you look at a meat-based dietary approach through the lens of a carnivore enthusiast, they will only include research making animal products look awesome and also highlight the disadvantages of plants-only.

These are both extremes in my opinion, and the truth is usually nestled somewhere in between. The great thing about the strategies I am going to show you is that you can use the style of eating that best fits you. Some probably will do better with more or less meat products. That is for you to discover. I want you to start looking at the nutrients you are consuming and when you are consuming them to fuel your training. For now, don't stress about the style.

METABOLIC FLEXIBILITY

Instead our goal is efficiency. You want your body to be able to use different macronutrients to support activity depending on what you are doing. Metabolic flexibility can be defined as "an adaptive response of an organism's metabolism to maintain energy homeostasis by maintaining fuel availability and demand during periods of fasting, varying meal composition, physical activity, and environmental fluctuations." (Reuben et. al., 2018)

Our bodies need to sense, traffic, store, and utilize substrates or macro-nutrients, like carbohydrates, fats, and proteins. We each have differing capacities to do these different things. You might see some individuals who can just eat whatever they want and never gain a pound. We chalk this up to being younger or having a higher metabolism. While there is some truth to that, the main difference is metabolic flexibility.

When we flood our body with too much food too often, a host of issues follow. If we look at it in terms of energy production, you would think that if there is more fuel in the tank, we will have more energy. But you know this isn't true. You have probably had a few times where you just ate too much and all you wanted to do was lie down for a while. We've all been there. It is not a lack of fuel leading to this lack of energy.

Instead tiny molecules in our cells are having an issue. These are our mitochondria. You may remember mitochondria from high school biology. -- the so-called power plants of our cells. This is where aerobic energy production occurs so you can do all the things you need to do.

The cool thing about these organelles, is they can use fat, carbs, and protein to produce energy for our body. This is the key for metabolic flexibility. When you have more and healthier mitochondria, you can create energy more easily. But when there is a large influx of substrates, like carbohydrates, it actually slows down the activity of the mitochondria.

This leads to assuming a ketogenic or high-fat/low-carb diet is the way to go. But the research indicates that when you have too much of any one nutrient, metabolic flexibility slows. So the key is balance and timing of your food to enhance this process.

There are a few things that can either speed up or slow down metabolic flexibility. We will focus on the ones you have direct control over. Since we are talking about nutrition here, we will spend most of our time discussing how to manipulate your eating to maximize the mitochondrial health in your cells.

Before we dive into the food, let's at least cover some simple things you can do to improve mitochondria biogenesis, or creating more mitochondria in your cells. We can be brief here because we have already touched on much of this throughout the book.

First, sleep is going to be crucial. When you disrupt your sleep/wake cycle or circadian rhythm, it causes issues. There is substantial evidence that those that follow a night shift work schedule are much more likely to be obese and develop associated metabolic disease. Not just those that have an altered day and night sleep/wake cycle -- but anyone who has sleep issues is more likely to suffer from disease, obesity, metabolic syndrome, cognitive impairment, and reduced metabolic flexibility. So, make sure you are doing the best you can to follow your optimal sleep schedule.

Next, there is cold exposure, a topic we've discussed previously. On top of the nervous system benefits of cold exposure, there is evidence that regular exposure to cold temperatures can increase metabolic flexibility. This is primarily achieved through the activation of brown fat adipose tissue. Brown fat is more metabolically active and will help utilize more energy to maintain energy balance.

Then, we can discuss nutritional implementations to improve metabolic flexibility. Chronic inflammation has been shown to not only increase risk for certain diseases, it also reduces flexibility. A good place to start on the nutrition side of the equation is with an anti-inflammatory diet.

Inflammation is a term that gets thrown around, but not everyone understands what it means. Inflammation is not a bad thing. This is a natural process that occurs in our body. When inflammation occurs, it signals your immune system to respond and heal the problem.

The issue we should be worried about is low-grade chronic inflammation. This is when your body is consistently sending signals of inflammation around the entire body. This is what leads to plaque buildup in arteries and other metabolic conditions, and, as mentioned, slows metabolic flexibility.

Hopefully, you are getting yearly blood work done. Inflammation can be detected by elevated proteins like C-reactive Protein and Tumor Necrosis Factor a. Regardless if you have chronic inflammation, these recommendations will still be good, but it increases the priority if proinflammatory markers are high.

It only makes sense to start here. Before we get into too many higher-level nutritional strategies, let's at least focus on the quality of food. First, you will eliminate foods that are the most likely to cause inflammation. We will review a list below. The results will not surprise you. In addition to avoiding inflammatory foods, you will include foods that help fight inflammation. And you will include foods that help restore a healthy microbiome. When the gut wall is damaged, the result will be an inflammatory response. We want to heal this the best we can to boost the overall process.

There are a number of anti-inflammatory diets out there like the DASH Diet and Mediterranean Diet. There is no one-size-fits-all approach here. Instead focus on the foods that generally promote an anti-inflammatory effect and avoid those that are proinflammatory.

Researchers have created a Dietary Inflammatory Index to help show which foods create a higher or lower inflammatory response. This may be a nice tool to help guide you along the way. According to this research, here are some of the top inflammatory foods to probably avoid.

- Processed Meats
- Refined grains
- Fast Food
- Margarine
- Trans Fats
- Sugar
- Vegetable Oil

There are many foods that fight inflammation. Here are some of the best options to regularly include in your diet.

- Poly unsaturated fats (Omega 3's)
- High Fiber Foods
- Fruits and Vegetables
- Olive oil
- Fatty fish
- Green leafy vegetables
- Tomatoes

For more on this you can check out Dr. Weil's Anti-inflammatory food pyramid for a good guide on what types of foods to consume.

But these should not shock you. Eat more real whole foods and limit heavily processed foods. You hopefully already know this, but if you don't have this down, everything else we talk about will be less effective. So your first step is to improve food quality by following an anti-inflammatory diet.

Once you are regularly eating these types of foods, there are training protocols that will be effective for enhancing metabolic flexibility. All the training programs discussed in this book will enhance metabolic flexibility in some manner. Interval training, long distance aerobic training, and resistance training all play roles.

We can boost the effects even more with the combination of dietary strategy and training. The crucial takeaway I want you to remember is this: not every day will require the same nutrient intake. When most people see a meal plan or calorie goal, it is often a single number. Maybe you were told you need to be eating 2,000 calories per day.

But the problem is, this is an average number. Think about your weekly routine. Do you do the same exact thing every day? Maybe you have a similar activity level at work each day. Maybe you sit most of the day during the week and then are more active on the weekend. But there is a good chance that each day is a little different.

Your training will look this way too. Some days you will train at higher intensity and some at lower intensity. You may even have a day where you do both a morning and evening session. Your fueling will now reflect the need you have to support your activity. This will take some time to plan and get used to, but I will share some simple ways to start eating this way.

For the first strategy, we will take more of a macro approach (pardon the pun), looking at the foods you take in for the day based on the type of training you have planned. To simplify this, try and organize your days into:

- Light to no exercise
- Moderate exercise
- Intense exercise

Based on this we can manipulate your total calories for the day and the amount of macronutrients you should consume.

To help you get started, days that you perform no exercise, light yoga or recovery sessions, or low intensity aerobic runs, you will categorize as light. Days that you perform strength training sessions or more zone 2 runs we will categorize into moderate, and anything in zone 3 or days with double sessions we will categorize as intense training. This should be a good start for you.

Now you will plan out your total calories and amount of macronutrient intake. There are many calculators out there that will give you an idea of these numbers. Keep in mind, these are estimates. They will not be perfect numbers. But they give you a good starting point and something to start tracking. Then you can adjust as needed.

Precision Nutrition has a free calculator you can use to get started. Visit the link here to get your personal numbers: https://www.precisionnutrition.com/nutrition-calculator. You can also check out a free calculator here: https://tdeecalculator.net/. Remember this will be our average number of total calories. Each day will be slightly different based on the type and amount of training you will be performing.

When we look at our different training day categories, we can start to look at our nutritional needs for those days. Based on the physiology discussed earlier in this book, you know that lower intensity training requires more fat utilization and higher intensity training requires more carbohydrate. This is the flexibility we are looking for. We want your body to use fat for fueling your training for as long as possible. Then when the intensity gets high enough, you can switch over to using more and more carbohydrates.

To help improve this flexibility, consume the foods that you want to use for fuel to support those workouts. Whatever fuels are present, the body will learn to use. If you primarily are eating carbs in your diet, no matter what style of training you are doing, your body will become more and more efficient at using those carbs. And when you stop eating carbs as much, guess what happens? Your body will rebel, and you will have cravings and even a decrease in performance.

Keep this in mind depending on what your current diet looks like. If this is a big change it might be a challenge at first. You may even experience lower energy. This will pass. Just be consistent and trust the process. You will notice a huge difference once you have given your body a chance to adapt.

WHAT A DAY LOOKS LIKE

Now, let's look at what your days will look like. Here is where it can get tricky when we start breaking down numbers. I will start with the numbers, if you are someone who really likes to track everything, but I will also share, hopefully a more practical way to set this up. Either way it will take planning and testing to find the best approach for you.

If you found your daily calorie goal already, we will start with that. Just remember this is an average and it will not be exactly the same each day. Some days will be slightly higher and some lower. But it is a good starting point to figure out a few numbers to work with.

We know our three macronutrients are fats, carbohydrates, and proteins, so these are the numbers we will focus on. Remember if you are following the anti-inflammatory pyramid, you should be getting high quality, whole foods and you should be getting your micronutrients sufficiently. For each of the days you will keep your protein relatively consistent at approximately 1 gram of protein per pound of body weight. If you weigh 170 pounds you would aim for 170 grams per day. This may seem like a higher number, but since you are active and training most days a week, we will need this protein to help support recovery.

For someone following a 2000 calorie daily intake, this amount of protein would be 680 calories or 34% of your nutrient intake. The rest of the calories will come from your carbohydrates and fats. Let's look at fat next.

Fat and protein intake will stay similar for each day. On your lower intensity days, we can slightly increase your fat intake since you will be using more fats for fuel on those days. Looking at the big picture, roughly 20-to-30% of your diet should consist of fats. Higher-intensity days we can drop closer to 20% and low-intensity days raise it up to 30%. With our 2000 calorie daily intake, this means we will range from 400-600 calories from fat or 44-67 grams of fat each day.

With carbs we will want to hit a range depending on the day of training we are doing. This is where the most manipulation will come in. This is also where it gets tricky. What is exactly low-carb? Depending on whom you ask you will get different definitions. A ketogenic diet, for example, would involve no more than 50 grams of carbs per day. For our purposes this may be too low to maintain training.

Yes, there are many athletes who can do this and benefit, but it is difficult to do and takes a long time to adapt to it. We know our brains need roughly 150 grams of carbohydrates per day to function properly. When you drop below this, unless you are adapted to ketones, you will experience side effects like dizziness, brain fog, confusion, and other problems. This number is an average, so it will not be exactly this number, but in the vicinity. If you want to experiment with the ketogenic approach, then you will have to get below this threshold of carb intake consistently. Otherwise just dipping down every few days may cause more damage than good.

Your goal will be to arrive at around 150 grams per day on your light or rest days. Depending on your size and need this number may be more or less. So experiment. On your moderate days aim for about 150-to-250 grams of carbohydrate and intense days aim for 250-to-350 grams. See the chart below for a complete layout of all the different macronutrient amounts for our example.

Day	Total	Protein (g)	Protein (cal)	Protein (%)	Fat (g)	Fat (cal)	Fat (%)	Carbs (g)	Carbs (cal)	Carbs (%)
Light/Rest	1700cal	170	680	40	57	510	30	128	510	30
Moderate	2000cal	170	680	34	55	500	25	205	820	41
Intense	2300cal	170	680	30	51	460	20	288	1160	50

Now, how do you implement all of this? Right now, you probably eat a relatively consistent diet. To start, you will need to track your food for at least a week. Longer is better, but let's start with a week. Then we can see how close or far you are from these numbers. Then you can see what you will have to manipulate.

From there, using the foods that you enjoy eating already (and on the approved anti-inflammatory list) start to create your own template. You will want a high-, moderate-, and low-carb day based on your numbers. Your low-carb day will consist primarily of no fruits, grains, pasta, or other high-carb foods. You will stick with vegetables, fats, and proteins for the day. Your moderate days will include 1-to-2 servings of extra carbohydrates. And your intense days will include 2-3 extra servings of carbs.

Once you understand your template, you can start filling in with different foods within those categories. In the beginning it helps to be consistent and repeat foods until you feel comfortable exploring other options.

ADVANCED STRATEGIES

Now if you can increase the quality of your food and get the basics behind the carbohydrate cycling, you are way ahead of most people out there. There are a few other strategies that can help improve your metabolic flexibility even more. Now we will focus on two specific tactics looking at the timing of your food intake.

FASTED EXERCISE

Fasted exercise has been a practice for varying reasons. With the increased popularity of intermittent fasting, we have seen an explosion in this trend. Remember the goal of what we are trying to accomplish: Increase the number of mitochondria and increase their function to produce energy more efficiently.

A study in 2013 compared exercise in a low-glycogen state versus normal-glycogen state. When you eat your body will convert the food into glucose to use for energy, but also to store glucose as glycogen so it has energy to use later. When you fast or exercise, you will decrease your glycogen stores. As soon as you eat again your body will repeat the process.

Researchers looked specifically at what happened to the mitochondria in these athletes when they performed exercise with either normal glycogen levels or low levels. They found subjects that performed exercise in the low-glycogen state were able to increase mitochondrial levels by three times compared to those with normal glycogen levels. This is an incredible increase.

As I previously mentioned, one way to reduce glycogen stores is to not eat. The drawback is there will be less energy to perform a tough workout. So, this strategy is solely for low-intensity, aerobic training style workouts. We will train your body to increase mitochondria so it can utilize fats better. Training here should solely be performed in the Zone 1 or 2 levels only.

Ideally these workouts are performed first thing in the morning. If this is not an option, you will want to wait around 6-8 hours after a meal to get the most benefit out of this type of training. Once you have completed your workout you can eat to refill your low glycogen stores and start to prepare for your next workout.

SLEEP LOW

This is essentially the same strategy, but with an added boost. It is more advanced and requires much more planning to accomplish. You will have to consider two days of eating and training for this tactic.

In 2016 a group of researchers compared the sleep low method to a control group. In this study, both groups ate the same amount of carbohydrates and performed the same type of training. The only difference was when the two groups ate their carbohydrates.

The sleep low group would perform a high intensity training session in the afternoon or evening, followed by a carbohydrate restriction. Once they finished the training session, they could still eat for the rest of the evening, but no carbohydrates were allowed. The following morning, in a fasted state, they performed another low-intensity training bout. After this session they could refuel with carbohydrates, until the next hard training session. This training program lasted for three weeks.

This study found the sleep low group saw greater improvements in cycling efficiency. In particular, greater time cycling to exhaustion at supramaximal intensities (very high), and greater 10-kilometer performance. As an added benefit they also saw great reductions in body fat with no loss in lean muscle tissue.

These numbers are incredibly impressive. The best part is, they didn't change what they were eating, simply when they were eating with their training. So for this type of training to work you will have to perform your higher intensity training sessions in the evening and lower intensity training in the morning. And in between the two, you will restrict your carbs.

My goal for you reading this chapter was not to confuse you with numbers. It is surprisingly difficult to do, but hopefully you have stayed with me. Nutrition is such a complex topic and our body is incredibly complex. Plus, we are all different, so the same eating plan will not work for every person. This is why I stay away from specific dietary philosophies, like plant-based, paleo, keto, etc. Many of these will work for the right individual. Your goal is to experiment to see what works best for you.

The bottom line is you should feel your nutrition supporting your training and performance. If you feel energized during your workouts and consistently see improvements, then you are on the right track. If you are feeling sluggish and low on energy, then it is time to re-evaluate.

To leave you, here are the action steps you will take to start to implement these strategies.

1. Clean out your kitchen of foods that are higher processed and pro-inflammatory and replace with foods from the anti-inflammatory pyramid.

2. Start tracking your macronutrients using My Fitness Pal or other food journal.

3. Determine your total caloric need using the online calculator and determine your macronutrient breakdown for each training day.

4. Observe your current eating plan to see how you can best manipulate to hit your macronutrient goals.

5. Create High-, Moderate-, and Low-carb nutrition templates you can start to follow for each day.

6. Implement fasted, low-intensity training or perform the sleep low method to further see gains and improve flexibility.

Now that you made it through your nutrition you can make it through just about anything. But hopefully I didn't cloud your brain too much because next up we will dive into your mental training.

CHAPTER 9

MENTAL TRAINING

To be honest this was an add-on chapter after starting to write this book. Originally, I did not think I would include anything on mental training, because it wasn't something I had used much. But then after completing my first Ultra Beast (50 kilometers long with 60 obstacles), I realized how wrong I was.

You do not have to be taking on an ultra-type race to benefit from mental training. After talking with Alex Hutchinson, the author of Endurance, and doing more research on the topic, I begin to realize how beneficial mental training is for any race distance.

When you look at what Alex reported in his book, it is clear that our limiting factors are often not going to be our physical abilities. Our brain will often put the brakes on first. This is an important concept to understand.

In a way, the training we are currently doing is to delay reaching the point we need to tap into our mental reserve. You have probably felt the difference between your body giving up and your mind giving up. Really the main times you probably felt your body being your limiting factor is something like a muscle cramp. At this point your body, or at least muscle, is saying "no more." An injury would probably fall under this category as well. In extreme cases you might see ultra-endurance athletes, pass out or just unable to walk another step due to fatigue or even muscles completely tearing.

Most cases it is our mind that is stopping us. You might feel like your legs can't push on anymore, but your brain will tell you to stop before your body will. There are several studies in which researchers asked participants to work a muscle until they no longer can complete a rep of an exercise. Next they will electrically stimulate that same "fatigued" muscle and the muscle will still contract. This is a demonstration of how the body can continue -- but the mind is preventing it.

The more trained you get, the less effort you feel you are exerting for a given intensity. So our physical training will fuel our mental training by delaying when we need to bear down and use the mind to continue. But at some point, as the exertion and fatigue escalate, you will need to recruit your brain, and this is something you can train for.

While books have already been written on this topic, here are a few areas that you can easily incorporate into your regular routine to make a significant difference in your performance.

GETTING UNCOMFORTABLE

This might seem obvious, but you need to get yourself uncomfortable. This will mean different things for different people. For some just going to the gym would qualify as being uncomfortable. If you picked up this book, however, I have the feeling you need something more.

While working out in general will get you uncomfortable, this is probably a discomfort you enjoy. Yes, it's true: by virtue of reading a book on how to realize your potential for OCR, you are slightly disturbed and enjoy torturing yourself. Hence, you will need to seek out and incorporate ways to make yourself more uncomfortable with things you do not enjoy.

This could be exercising when you otherwise don't want to. Sometimes there are days our body is telling us to take a break and other when we just don't feel like doing it. You will need to understand the difference. If it is the latter, you will make it a point to seize the opportunity to build mental strength and get out there and get it done.

This might include times when conditions are not ideal. It might be pouring rain outside the day you have a long run planned, or maybe it is much colder or hotter than you like for your run. <u>These are the most important days for you to get out there.</u> No, it probably won't be a PR run for you, but that is not the point. The point is that you are doing something you prefer not to do.

Another simple way to do this that I often find myself recommending for clients, is taking cold showers. This has become a trendy thing to do and there are many benefits from it. For our discussion here, it is simply to get you doing something you probably don't enjoy doing. The key is to breathe through the discomfort and keep telling yourself it really isn't that bad. We will talk about self-talk in a bit, but for now just trust me on this one.

HAVE A MANTRA

According to Wikipedia, the definition of mantra is:

<u>A sacred utterance, a numinous sound, a syllable, work, or group of words believed to have psychological and/or spiritual powers.</u>

Something that has been practiced for thousands of years is -- in the latest neuroscience research to help quiet the mind and help focus -- starting to show benefits.

When you are in pain while racing, it is amazing how much benefit you can receive from using this practice. Even if we can't explain all the benefits with science, the simple fact of distraction will go a long way during some races.

As I was training for my Ultra Beast, I credit using a mantra for much of my success. Using a mantra gave me an extra tool to rely on when things got especially tough. I will admit, I am no expert in this area of sports psychology, but I would like to at least share some aspects of using a mantra that benefit myself as well as clients I have worked with.

A mantra can have meaning to you or can be meaningless. Sometimes it is using a word or words that are enjoyable to say. Personally, I chose something that had meaning to me. It took me some time to come up with it. During my training I would let my mind wander and find things that helped pick me up when I was struggling. There are certain things you can tell yourself or picture in your head that give you a boost of energy or simply put you in a better place.

To help get you started, think about what your limiting factor is on your body during a race. Maybe your legs get heavy or your grip gives out. Think about that area that you wish would improve. Now imagine how it would feel if, suddenly, your weakness was now your strength. Your legs were as light as a feather or you had bone-crushing grip. How do you feel now? Is there a word or phase that can capture that feeling?

This is a great starting point to help develop your own personal mantra. Acknowledge your weakness and turn it to a strength.

POSITIVE SELF-TALK

This may make no sense to you right now, but I have to say it anyway. You are not your thoughts. This is a difficult concept to explain in a few short paragraphs and is covered more deeply in the books The 7 Habits of Highly Effective Individuals and Untethered Soul. If you want to go down that rabbit hole, I recommend both those readings.

The idea is this: Those voices you hear in your head are not you. They are a piece of your subconscious trying to control you. Understanding this, you can use those voices to help you or hurt you. The decision is entirely up to you and no one else.

You may have heard of the Old Cherokee story of the boy asking his elder for advice about an internal battle he is struggling with. He is told that there is a battle of two wolves going on inside him and every other person. One wolf is evil. He is anger, envy, sorrow, regret, greed, arrogance, self-pity, guilt, resentment, inferiority, and ego. The other wolf is good. He is joy, peace, love, hope, serenity, humility, kindness, truth, faith, and compassion.

When the boy asks which wolf will win, the old Cherokee replies, "The one you feed."

Hopefully this story hits home for you. You are in control of every thought in your head. While they may seem harmless at first, these thoughts will manifest into actions in some form. They will have real-life impacts. Simple words like, "I'm tired," or "I can't do this" will become self-fulfilling prophecies.

Your first step is to be aware of when these negative thoughts start to creep into your head. When you are aware you can acknowledge them, you can deliberately start to increase positive self-talk. Research has even shown what a dramatic impact this can make on physical performance.

A 2014 study observed 24 active men and women, and the impact of deliberate positive self-talk. They were divided into two groups. One group received self-talk coaching and the other did not. After two weeks the group who received the positive self-talk coaching had a lower rating of perceived exertion and a longer time to exhaustion by almost two minutes.

These are incredible results. With no other training than positive self-talk, the athletes felt like their effort was getting easier and they lasted two minutes longer in a time trial to failure. Imagine if you could push another two minutes when everyone else was giving up.

The final point I wanted to bring up on this idea of self talk I learned from Mental Performance Coach Brian Cain. This simple statement completely changed how I viewed self talk. You must always talk to yourself and never listen to yourself.

I know this might sound strange, but think about it. When you are listening to yourself, it tends to be reactive. That little voice inside your head starts telling you something. Rarely does this voice scream, "You can do this!" Instead it whispers, this is too hard, you should quit, you won't finish, etc.

But talking to yourself is proactive. You have complete control over this. Using the strategies mentioned above you can control the conversation and turn it into a positive motivator. Usually with social interactions we need to listen more and talk less. But when dealing with your internal dialogue YOU have the drive the conversation. You need to talk more and listen less.

ENJOY THE VIEW

I joked with a few clients, training for my Ultra, that if I could make it an hour on my treadmill for a run, then I could easily handle a 30-mile OCR. While that might be a slight exaggeration, I do believe there is some truth in that.

We often are looking for the most comfortable way to get through things. I mentioned this earlier about getting comfortable being uncomfortable. During training, we often use distractions and external motivations to help us through the workouts. This might be listening to your favorite music during a run or just picking a scenic route to enjoy the view.

These are all great things to use at times. But often we become reliant on these external motivators. When you are in the race, you are on your own. The longer the distance the more you will be alone with your thoughts. Hopefully you have been training your positive thoughts and this is easy for you to do. But you must put yourself in that situation.

Here is a picture of my view when running on our treadmill. It is an incredibly exciting wall I know. But sometimes, I get on the treadmill and go. It will seem like agony. <u>That is the point</u>. Don't cover up the clock and no music is allowed. Just you, your thoughts, and the wall. This might seem silly, but I promise this will get you strong. This may even turn into your own form of meditation.

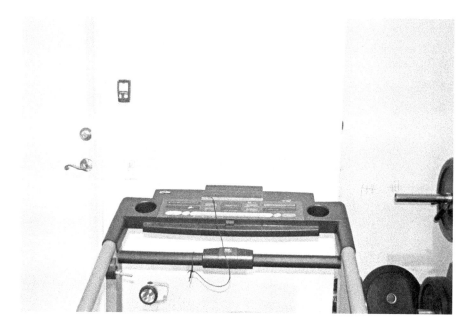

GET SHIT DONE

I have previously mentioned Dan John in this book. I once heard him present at a conference a few years back and he brought up a concept that was incredibly simple yet insightful. The idea was shark habits.

The idea is simple, one bite and it is gone. Just like a shark. There are things in our life that clutter us up. Often little things that we just don't want to do. This could be doing dishes, answering an email, making a phone call, taking out the trash, etc. An annoying but necessary task presents itself: Do it now and have it over. That's a shark habit.

This may sound like it has nothing to do with the topic of mental toughness, but when racing you are going to have to do a lot of things you really may not want to do. Get used to this feeling. This does not have to involve training at all. Anytime in your life you have something that can get done with "one bite" you will do it right then. No making lists or putting it off. Just do it and be done with it.

The more you practice the art of getting shit done the more productive you will be, and it will just be a new habit that you don't even think about. If something is in your way, you just take it on and get it done. The key is to be consistent. Get used to doing things you just don't feel like doing.

These are just a few simple things you can do on a regular basis to work on your mindset and mental toughness. If you want the total package, to get everything you can out of your training, you will need to devote time into both your mental and physical training on a regular basis.

CHAPTER 10

GET TO WORK

Throughout this book, I have provided everything you need for an incredibly comprehensive training and nutrition plan. You may have already started with some of the items discussed, which is awesome. Before we wrap things up, I want to leave you with a few action steps to help you get started.

PLAN OUT YOUR YEAR

It can be a challenge for many to think this far ahead. But if you truly want to see the benefits of your training you need to plan it all out. Pick one race that you would like to peak for. Then start working backwards. Depending on your starting point and how long of a race you are training for, your time will vary. For most races, 12 weeks is probably a good starting point.

Plan for one deload or recovery week for every three weeks of training you do. Then you can schedule out which days you will perform strength, running, and tactical workouts. When adding mileage to your running try not to add more than 10% total mileage per week.

DETERMINE YOUR BASELINE

We need to understand where you are starting from. This will help you chart the progress in your training and help you determine your major areas of weakness. We have discussed different assessments in this book extensively. Pick ones that will work best for you, but make sure you cover the primary training areas:

- Movement Quality
- Aerobic Capacity
- Strength
- Power
- Recovery

Once you have implemented a training plan, go back and check your work. If strength was your weakness, then you should have gotten stronger from your training. A simple concept but many just expect that any workouts will get you better. Only if it is the right workout will this improvement happen.

TRACK YOUR NUTRITION

There are just too many variables with nutrition to just guess at. You will have to put some work into this. Start tracking your food with a journal like My Fitness Pal. Keep your priority front and center. Are you trying to lose weight or boost performance? This will change your nutritional goals. If training for weight loss keep an eye on total calories. If you are trying to maximize performance, you will shift your attention to macro-nutrients and food quality.

Have a standard plan for each type of training. Remember which days you will want to increase carbohydrate intake and which days you want to decrease it. Pay attention to the timing of your food when appropriate as well. There is no perfect plan here. Do the best you can to be consistent so you can make educated decisions on how you should eat.

NETWORK WITH A MEDICAL PROFESSIONAL

Injuries do happen. My goal is that by following a system like this we can limit most injuries, but unfortunately, they can still pop up. If something comes up address it as soon as possible. And this does not mean posting online for suggestions on knee pain.

Find a professional in your area that can properly diagnose and treat your issues. Yes, this takes more time and investment, but it is the fastest way to recover. Just find someone that you trust and understands what you are trying to do. You can find great professionals in your area through this link. Just look for a SFMA-certified practitioner.

https://www.functionalmovement.com/members

GET SUPPORT

Why do this alone? Training partners and coaches can lead to dramatic improvements in your performance. I promise that you can take everything in this book, apply it, and get great results. But there is something about having another person keep you accountable.

If you have enjoyed reading this so far, you might be interested in checking out my Fuel and Fire Elite Program. This is a 90 day program designed to walk you through everything discussed in this book, plus more. Each week you will be given a lesson plan to follow.

This lesson plan will include your strength workouts, running workouts, tactical training, obstacle strategies, nutrition lessons, recovery lesson, and much more. Plus, you will get access to my private Facebook group where I can answer any questions and help you out along the way.

I am incredibly grateful that you have trusted me so far in purchasing and reading this book. My goal was to provide you more value than you paid for. I offer the same promise with any of my coaching programs. In fact, if you don't feel like you got everything you expected out of the program you can ask for a complete refund.

To access this program and receive special pricing for purchasing this book visit www.ocrunderground.com/book-bonus.

If you are still on the fence, I encourage you to go through the sample program outlined in the appendix of this book. This will be a great start for you. Then when you are ready to progress you can join the Fuel and Fire Elites.

Now, it is time to get to work. This book is all about taking action. You have the plan laid out. It is up to you to follow through. Just like most things that are truly worth it, you will get out what you put in. You took the first step in educating yourself on how to do this right. Now get out there and do it. I hope to see you at a future race. And if you ever need that extra support feel free to reach out to me.

APPENDIX

TRAINING PLAN

There are a variety of distances and types of obstacle course races you may be training for. With that in mind I wanted to create something to help you apply what you have learned in this book, so you can get started on the right track.

In the following pages you will find your jump start program for the next 4 weeks. This is your first phase of training that you will go through. You will find your running plan, strength program, and tactical training.

Follow the plan in a progressive manner. This means your first week will be easing into it. You won't be crushing it right off that bat. Instead, learn the movements, work on your running form and tracking your heart rate, and improving the quality of your work. Each week you will increase intensity. By the final week you are attempting a PR, or personal record, for each workout. When you start your next phase you start over, easing your way back in. This way you have built-in recovery weeks, so you aren't pushing too hard all the time.

In this plan you'll train for a 10k distance race. The first week is assuming you have some training background, but if you are brand new you may need to cut back on some of the distances.

The calendar is simply a guide to see how the program might be laid out for you. But make edits so it fits your schedule best. It will include 6 training days, but get as many days that fit your schedule. This is simply an ideal situation, but life doesn't always work out that way. And one final reminder, visit www.ocrunderground.com/book-bonus to printable workout logs and links to video demos for all exercises.

Enjoy!

28 Day Calendar

Fuel & Fire Training Calendar

	DAY 1	DAY 2	DAY 3	DAY 4	DAY 5	DAY 6	DAY 7
WEEK 1	AEROBIC RUN	STREGNTH WORKOUT A	FAST FINISH RUN	RECOVERY DAY	STRENGTH WORKOUT B	LONG INTERVAL RUN 1	TACTICAL WORKOUT
WEEK 2	RECOVERY DAY	AEROBIC RUN	STRENGTH WORKOUT A	FAST FINISH RUN	RECOVERY DAY	STRENGTH WORKOUT B	LONG INTERVAL RUN 1
WEEK 3	TACTICAL WORKOUT	RECOVERY DAY	AEROBIC RUN	STRENGTH WORKOUT A	HILL REPEATS	RECOVERY DAY	STRENGTH WORKOUT B
WEEK 4	LONG INTERVAL RUN 2	TACTICAL WORKOUT	RECOVERY DAY	AEROBIC RUN	STRENGTH WORKOUT A	HILL REPEATS	RECOVERY DAY

Running Program

Aerobic Run

Perform .5 miles in zone 1
3 miles in zone 2
.5 miles in zone 1
Progress by 10% each week.

Fast Finish Run

Perform 5 minutes in zone 1
25 minutes in zone 2
12 minutes in zone 3
5 minutes in zone 1

Long Interval Run 1

Perform 5 minutes in zone 1
5 minutes in zone 2
4 X 3 minutes in zone 3 w/ a 2 minute zone 1 recovery

Long Interval Run 2

Perform 5 minutes in zone 1
5 minutes in zone 2
3 X 5 minutes in zone 3 w/ a 2 minute zone 1 recovery

Hill Repeats

Perform 5 minutes in zone 1
5 minutes in zone 2
10 X 30 second uphill zone 3 sprints with a 90 second zone 1 recovery

Strength Workouts

WORKOUT A			Week1	Week2	Week3	Week4
Order / **Myofascial Release**	**Sets**	**Reps**				
1 Calves	1	60s				
2 Quads	1	60s				
3 Adductors	1	60s				
4 Hip Rotators	1	60s				
5 Lats	1	60s				
Order / **Mobility**	**Sets**	**Reps**	**Lbs**	**Lbs**	**Lbs**	**Lbs**
1 Crocodile Breathing	1	6br				
2 Toe/Heel Sitting	1	6br				
3 Brettzel 2.0	1	6br				
4 Anterior/Posterior Dynamic Hip	1	8ea				
5 Dowel Assisted Shoulder Stretch	1	8ea				
Order / **Stability/Correctives**	**Sets**	**Reps**	**Lbs**	**Lbs**	**Lbs**	**Lbs**
1 Single Leg Bridge	2	8ea				
2 Bird Dogs	2	4ea				
3 Band Pull Apart	2	10				
4 KB Marching	2	8ea				
Order / **Power Development**	**Sets**	**Reps**	**Lbs**	**Lbs**	**Lbs**	**Lbs**
A1 Power Step Jump	3	8ea				
A2 MB Half Kneeling Rotational Throw	3	8ea				
Order / **Resistance Training Exercises**	**Sets**	**Reps**	**Lbs**	**Lbs**	**Lbs**	**Lbs**
B1 KB Goblet Squat	3	12				
B2 Assisted Pull Ups	3	12				
C1 DB Reverse Lunge	3	10ea				
C2 Push Up	3	12				
D1 SB Hamstring Curls	3	12				
D2 USB Around The Word	3	6ea				
Order / **Conditioning**	**Sets**	**Reps**	**Lbs**	**Lbs**	**Lbs**	**Lbs**
E1 Tabata Circuit						
Mountain Climbers/MB Slams	4	20s				
Notes:						

WORKOUT B				Week1	Week2	Week3	Week4
Order	Myofascial Release	Sets	Reps				
1	Calves	1	60s				
2	Quads	1	60s				
3	Adductors	1	60s				
4	Hip Rotators	1	60s				
5	Lats	1	60s				
Order	Mobility	Sets	Reps	Lbs	Lbs	Lbs	Lbs
1	Crocodile Breathing	1	6br				
2	Toe/Heel Sitting	1	6br				
3	Brettzel 2.0	1	6br				
4	Anterior/Posterior Dynamic HIp	1	8ea				
5	Dowel Assisted Shoulder Stretch	1	8ea				
Order	Activation	Sets	Reps	Lbs	Lbs	Lbs	Lbs
1	Floor Slides	2	8				
2	Plank Hold	2	30s				
3	Half Kneeling Chops	2	8ea				
4	Toe Touch Squatting	2	8				
Order	Power Development	Sets	Reps	Lbs	Lbs	Lbs	Lbs
A1	KB Swings	3	10				
A2	BOSU Smash Push Up	3	6				
Order	Resistance Training Exercises	Sets	Reps	Lbs	Lbs	Lbs	Lbs
B1	KB Deadlift	3	12				
B2	Landmine Half Kneeling Press	3	10ea				
B3	Dead Hang	3	30s				
C1	DB Step Ups	3	10ea				
C2	DB Wide Stance Row	3	10ea				
C3	KB SA Farmer Carry	3	30s ea				
Order	Conditioning	Sets	Reps	Time	Time	Time	Time
D1	Assault Bike	1	2 miles				
	Bike sub 1 Mile Run						

Notes:

Tactical Workout				Week1	Week2	Week3	Week4
Order	Myofascial Release	Sets	Reps				
1	Calves	1	60s				
2	Quads	1	60s				
3	Adductors	1	60s				
4	Hip Rotators	1	60s				
5	Lats	1	60s				
Order	Active Warm Up	Sets	Reps	Lbs	Lbs	Lbs	Lbs
1	Brettzel	1	5br				
2	Spiderman Stretch	1	8ea				
3	Leg Lowering	1	8ea				
4	Push Up To Downward Dog	1	8				
5	Knee Hugs	1	8ea				
6	Quad Stretch	1	6ea				
7	A Skips	1	8ea				
8	B Skips	1	8ea				
9	Backpedal	1	8ea				
10	Side Shuffle	1	6				
Order	Circuit 1	Sets	Reps	Lbs	Lbs	Lbs	Lbs
A1	DB Walking Lunges	3	10ea				
A2	Bear Crawl	3	10ea				
A3	Switch Grip	3	5ea				
Order	Circuit 2	Sets	Reps	Lbs	Lbs	Lbs	Lbs
B1	Run	4	90s				
B2	Bucket Carry	4	60s				
B3	Box Jumps	4	6				
B4	Lateral Bear Crawl	4	10ea				
B5	Hanging Marching	4	8ea				
B6	Burpees	4	8				
Order	Conditioning	Sets	Reps	Time	Time	Time	Time

Notes:

WORKS CITED

Alwyn Cosgrove, and Craig Rasmussen. *Secrets of Successful Program Design : A How-to Guide for Busy Fitness Professionals*. Champaign, Il, Human Kinetics, 2021.

Boyle, Michael. *Advances in Functional Training*. Lotus Publishing Chicester, 2010.

Fitzgerald, Matt. *80/20 Running : Run Stronger And Race Faster By Training Slower*. New York, New York, Nal, New American Library, 2014.

Gray Cook. *Movement: Functional Movement Systems - Screening, Assessment, Corrective s*. Lotus Publishing, 2011.

Hutchison, Amy T., and Leonie K. Heilbronn. "Metabolic Impacts of Altering Meal Frequency and Timing – Does When We Eat Matter?" *Biochimie*, vol. 124, May 2016, pp. 187–197, 10.1016/j.biochi.2015.07.025. Accessed 18 Dec. 2019.

John, Dan. "Strength Standards...Sleepless in Seattle." *Dan John*, 13 Apr. 2013, danjohn.net/2013/04/strength-standards-sleepless-in-seattle/. Accessed 13 Oct. 2020.

Kiecolt-Glaser, Janice K. "Stress, Food, and Inflammation: Psychoneuroimmunology and Nutrition at the Cutting Edge." *Psychosomatic Medicine*, vol. 72, no. 4, May 2010, pp. 365–369, 10.1097/psy.0b013e3181dbf489. Accessed 19 Oct. 2019.

MARQUET, LAURIE-ANNE, et al. "Enhanced Endurance Performance by Periodization of Carbohydrate Intake." *Medicine & Science in Sports & Exercise*, vol. 48, no. 4, Apr. 2016, pp. 663–672, insights. ovid.com/medicine-science-sports-exercise/mespex/2016/04/000/ enhanced-endurance-performance-periodization/11/00005768, 10.1249/mss.0000000000000823. Accessed 28 July 2019.

Minihane, Anne M., et al. "Low-Grade Inflammation, Diet Composition and Health: Current Research Evidence and Its Translation." *British Journal of Nutrition*, vol. 114, no. 7, 31 July 2015, pp. 999–1012, www.ncbi.nlm. nih.gov/pmc/articles/PMC4579563/, 10.1017/s0007114515002093.

Mooventhan, A, and L Nivethitha. "Scientific Evidence-Based Effects of Hydrotherapy on Various Systems of the Body." *North American Journal of Medical Sciences*, vol. 6, no. 5, 2014, p. 199, 10.4103/1947-2714.132935.

Niklas Psilander. *The Effect of Different Exercise Regimens on Mitochondrial Biogenesis and Performance*. Stockholm, Karolinska Institutet, 2014.

Psilander, Niklas, et al. "Exercise with Low Glycogen Increases PGC-1α Gene Expression in Human Skeletal Muscle." *European Journal of Applied Physiology*, vol. 113, no. 4, 2 Oct. 2012, pp. 951–963, 10.1007/ s00421-012-2504-8. Accessed 13 Oct. 2020.

Shivappa, Nitin, et al. "Designing and Developing a Literature-Derived, Population-Based Dietary Inflammatory Index." *Public Health Nutrition*, vol. 17, no. 8, 1 Aug. 2014, pp. 1689–1696, pubmed.ncbi.nlm.nih. gov/23941862/, 10.1017/S1368980013002115. Accessed 20 Sept. 2020.

Smith, Reuben L, et al. "Metabolic Flexibility as an Adaptation to Energy Resources and Requirements in Health and Disease." *Endocrine Reviews*, vol. 39, no. 4, 24 Apr. 2018, pp. 489–517, 10.1210/er.2017-00211.

Wiewelhove, Thimo, et al. "A Meta-Analysis of the Effects of Foam Rolling on Performance and Recovery." *Frontiers in Physiology*, vol. 10, 9 Apr. 2019, 10.3389/fphys.2019.00376.

Wikipedia Contributors. "Hero's Journey." *Wikipedia*, Wikimedia Foundation, 8 Oct. 2020, en.wikipedia.org/wiki/Hero%27s_journey# Summary. Accessed 13 Oct. 2020.

Zarrinpar, Amir, et al. "Daily Eating Patterns and Their Impact on Health and Disease." *Trends in Endocrinology & Metabolism*, vol. 27, no. 2, Feb. 2016, pp. 69–83, 10.1016/j.tem.2015.11.007.

CPSIA information can be obtained
at www.ICGtesting.com
Printed in the USA
BVHW041049220221
600778BV00009B/1139